T0210176

Behavioral Health

Editor

MEAGAN W. VERMEULEN

PRIMARY CARE:
CLINICS IN OFFICE PRACTICE

www.primarycare.theclinics.com

Consulting Editor
JOEL J. HEIDELBAUGH

March 2023 • Volume 50 • Number 1

ELSEVIER

1600 John F. Kennedy Boulevard • Suite 1800 • Philadelphia, Pennsylvania, 19103-2899

http://www.theclinics.com

PRIMARY CARE: CLINICS IN OFFICE PRACTICE Volume 50, Number 1
March 2023 ISSN 0095-4543, ISBN-13: 978-0-323-93943-0

Editor: Taylor Hayes
Developmental Editor: Jessica Cañaberal

Primary Care: Clinics in Office Practice (ISSN: 0095-4543) is published quarterly by Elsevier Inc., 360 Park Avenue South, New York, NY 10010-1710. Months of issue are March, June, September, and December. Periodicals postage paid at New York, NY and additional mailing offices. Subscription prices are $277.00 per year (US individuals), $629.00 (US institutions), $100.00 (US students), $321.00 (Canadian individuals), $712.00 (Canadian institutions), $100.00 (Canadian students), $379.00 (international individuals), $712.00 (international institutions), and $175.00 (international students). Foreign air speed delivery is included in all *Clinics* subscription prices. All prices are subject to change without notice. POSTMASTER: Send address changes to *Primary Care: Clinics in Office Practice*, Elsevier Periodicals Customer Service, 11830 Westline Industrial Drive, St. Louis, MO 63146. Customer Service Health Sciences Division, Subscription Customer Service, 3251 Riverport Lane, Maryland Heights, MO 63043. **Customer Service: 1-800-654-2452 (U.S. and Canada); 314-447-8871 (outside U.S. and Canada). Fax: 314-447-8029. E-mail: journalscustomerservice-usa@elsevier.com (for print support); journalsonlinesupport-usa@elsevier.com (for online support).**

Reprints. For copies of 100 or more, of articles in this publication, please contact the Commercial Reprints Department, Elsevier Inc., 360 Park Avenue South, New York, NY 10010-1710. Tel. 212-633-3874; Fax: 212-633-3820; E-mail: reprints@elsevier.com.

Primary Care: Clinics in Office Practice is covered in *MEDLINE/PubMed (Index Medicus)* and *EMBASE/Excerpta Medica, Current Contents/Clinical Medicine,* and *ISI/BIOMED.*

Contributors

CONSULTING EDITOR

JOEL J. HEIDELBAUGH, MD, FAAFP, FACG
Clinical Professor, Departments of Family Medicine and Urology, Director of Medical
Student Education and Clerkship Director, Department of Family Medicine, University of
Michigan Medical School, Ann Arbor, Michigan; Ypsilanti Health Center, Ypsilanti,
Michigan

EDITOR

MEAGAN W. VERMEULEN, MD, FAAFP
Founding Program Director, Inspira Family Medicine Residency Program, Mullica Hill,
New Jersey; Associate Professor, Department of Family Medicine, Rowan-Virtua School
of Osteopathic Medicine, Stratford, New Jersey

AUTHORS

COURTNEY BARRY, PsyD, MS
Assistant Professor, Department of Psychiatry and Behavioral Medicine, Medical College
of Wisconsin, Milwaukee, Wisconsin

BENJAMIN A. BENSADON, EdM, PhD
SIMEDHealth, Gainesville, Florida

JAMES MICHAEL M. BRENNAN, PhD
San Francisco VA Healthcare System, San Francisco, California

JENNIFER CACERES, MD
Associate Professor of Medicine, Florida Atlantic University, Schmidt College of Medicine,
Boca Raton, Florida

ANGELA L. COLISTRA, PhD, LPC, CAADC, CCS
Lehigh Valley Health Network Department of Family Medicine, Allentown, Pennsylvania;
Assistant Professor, University of South Florida Morsani College of Medicine, Tampa,
Florida

NINA CROWLEY, PhD, RD
Professional Affiliations & Education Manager, Medical Body Composition for Seca
Corporation, South Carolina

KAMINI GEER, MD, MPH
Program Director, AdventHealth East Orlando Family Medicine Residency, Clinical
Assistant Professor Dr. Kiran C., Orlando, Florida

CONSTANCE GUNDACKER, MD, MPH
Assistant Professor, Department of Pediatrics, Medical College of Wisconsin, Children's Corporate Center, Milwaukee, Wisconsin

ELIZABETH GUNDERSEN, MD, FHM, FAAHPM
Associate Professor of Hospice and Palliative Medicine, University of Colorado School of Medicine, Aurora, Colorado

KRISTA L. HERBERT, PhD
VA Portland Health Care System, Portland, Oregon

ALLISON HOLLEY, MD
Assistant Professor of Medicine, Florida Atlantic University Schmidt College of Medicine, Boca Raton, Florida

DANIEL J. MAJARWITZ, MD
PGY-3, Department of Psychiatry and Behavioral Medicine, East Carolina University, Greenville, North Carolina

BRANDYN MASON, DO, MSMED, MHSA
Associate Program Director Carle Health Family Medicine Residency, Assisstant Medical Director for Quality/Safety/Carle Experience for Primary Care, Carle Foundation Hospital, Urbana, Illinois

AMANDA MELLOWSPRING, MS, RD/N, CEDS-S
Vice President of Nutrition Services, Monte Nido & Affiliates, Miami, Florida

ROBIN NEWBURN, DO
Assistant Clinical Professor of Primary Care Medicine, Ohio University Heritage College of Osteopathic Medicine, Dublin, Ohio

PARVATHI PERUMAREDDI, DO
Associate Professor of Family Medicine, Department of Medicine, Florida Atlantic University, Schmidt College of Medicine, Boca Raton, Florida

JOANNA PETRIDES, MBS, PsyD
Professor, Department of Family Medicine, Assistant Professor, Department of Psychology, Rowan-Virtua School of Osteopathic Medicine, Stratford, New Jersey

ERIN SMITH, DO
Lehigh Valley Health Network Department of Family Medicine, Allentown, Pennsylvania; Assistant Professor, University of South Florida Morsani College of Medicine, Tampa, Florida; Neighborhood Centers of the Lehigh Valley, Allentown, Pennsylvania

ANDREA WARD, DO
Lehigh Valley Health Network Department of Family Medicine, Allentown, Pennsylvania; LVPG Family Medicine-Hamburg, Lehigh Valley Health Network, Hamburg, Pennsylvania

TABATHA WELLS, MD, FAAFP
Mahomet, Illinois

Contents

> Primary-care settings have a unique advantage to reaching a broad range of the population and the ability to address a wide array of presenting problems, including substance-use. With high rates of substance-use in the United States and low rates of substance-use treatment utilization, the primary-care office is key in assessing and supporting patients in changing substance-use behaviors. Motivational interviewing is a conversational tool physicians can use to highlight intrinsic motivation for change and support specific changes patients want to make. Providers can also apply motivational interviewing to a variety of chronic health care behaviors.

> Stepped-care (SC) models have been adopted in primary care settings as a method for treating mental health conditions within primary care. In a SC model, a patient's symptoms are assessed, and an intervention is prescribed that matches the severity of symptoms. Thus, the SC model offers a variety of steps and levels of treatment that range from low to high intensity. Progression in treatment is monitored on a weekly basis and patients are stepped up or down in level of care depending on their clinical response to the intervention.

> Attention-deficit hyperactivity disorder is a neurodevelopmental disorder involving dysregulation of multiple neural circuits, manifesting in symptoms such as inattention, impulsivity, and hyperactivity. Diagnosis requires onset of symptoms before age 12 years. However, symptoms often persist

throughout lifetime, although they may change over time. The Diagnostic and Statistical Manual of Mental Disorders Fifth Edition formally lists the clinical criteria. Management involves pharmacologic agents, such as stimulant and/or nonstimulant medications, and providers should monitor closely for any adverse effects. Nonpharmacologic interventions may be implemented and can be used in conjunction with pharmacotherapy, although medications should be at the forefront of treatment.

Social media and technology use has increased over the past several years. Inappropriate use or overuse of social media and internet can lead to increase in mental health disorders. Primary care physicians should screen adolescents and young adults for social media and technology use and cyberbullying using a screening tool developed for healthcare settings. Parents should be educated on keeping open lines of communications with their teens to help navigate appropriate technology behaviors and put proper boundaries in place. Counseling interventional programs and educational programs can be utilized to help prevent cyberbullying and treat those who have been affected.

Mental health disorders in college students are an increasing concern within the United States. Many factors lead to the increase in disorders during this transition period but most are centered on the needed adjustments into adult life and lack of foundation to make these changes. Socioeconomic and racial demographics play a role in the risks of developing and seeking treatment of these issues. Mental health first aid may become the first-line modality to finding and treating mental health disorders in these students.

This chapter discusses the barriers related to treating substance use disorders (SUD) in primary-care building an argument that stigma is the largest health disparity left to overcome in this setting. Reviewing the history of treatment in primary-care, common medications prescribed, laws, and regulations that make this care possible in this setting. Owing to the sheer numbers of people with SUD and mental health concerns, primary-care and their related payers must recognize for many regions of the United States those community needs are related to the diagnosis and treatment of SUDs and their related behavioral and physical health problems.

Trauma is common within the United States. It is important for individuals to understand how trauma may affect their health and how trauma in childhood can have adverse effects on a child's development and health. To reduce retraumatization of patients, it is imperative to use trauma-informed approaches in a clinical encounter. Screening can be an effective way to understand a patient's trauma history. When screening for trauma, it is important to take a family-centered approach and provide appropriate referrals if a patient screens positive for trauma. Primary care providers are essential players in addressing and preventing trauma.

Adjustment disorder is a disorder characterized by an extreme emotional reaction to a stressor. It is defined diagnostically with either the Diagnostic and Statistical Manual V or ICD-11 definitions. There is currently a diagnostic tool that is still being validated to assist with diagnosing adjustment disorder. The prevalence of this disorder ranges from 0.2% to 40%, depending on the stressful circumstances that the patient experiences. There are several treatments available for adjustment disorder, ranging from psychological interventions, natural therapies to pharmacotherapies.

Stigma and bias surrounding body weight is both explicit and implicit, but the most concerning impact on individuals is internalized stigma which is correlated with poor physical and mental health. Strategies to combat this public health concern include increasing awareness, education around the complex disease of obesity, proper use of communication and language surrounding weight, health, and treatment approaches, addressing equipment and practices in the clinical environment, and larger, systemic approaches to policy. Addressing stigma for a condition impacting the majority of our population is critical for the best health and well-being of our patients and ourselves.

Eating disorders are mental health disorders with complicating medical, psychiatric, and nutritional comorbidities. Common eating disorder diagnoses include anorexia nervosa, bulimia nervosa, binge eating disorder, avoidant restrictive food intake disorder, and other specified feeding or eating disorder. Unspecified feeding or eating disorder is most applicable in brief acute care settings. Eating disorders occur across age, gender, racial, ethnic, and socioeconomic variables. Effective assessment, intervention, and collaborative treatment are needed to decrease risk factors and increase opportunities for recovery.

Mental health is a very important component of whole health because the body, mind, and spirit are woven together to create the fabric of a person's life. Many people in the United States and globally are living with mental health challenges, and it seems that much more attention has been given to anxiety-related mental health conditions in the past few years due to the coronavirus disease 2019 pandemic. The pandemic may certainly have accelerated the onset of mental health conditions for some who were already predisposed, whether it be to depression, anxiety, psychosis, or obsessive-compulsive disorder, to name a few.

Perinatal mood disorders are a leading cause of disability worldwide and suicide is a leading cause of maternal death in the first year after giving birth. The three categories of perinatal mood disorders are postpartum blues, postpartum depression, and postpartum psychosis. Identifying risk factors may allow clinicians to provide patients with interventions to potentially prevent development of these disorders. Universal screening for perinatal mood disorders can lead to earlier identification and treatment. Collaborative care methods, incorporating the entire family into treatment, therapy service, and providing support services are recommended as first-line intervention strategies before moving on to pharmacologic management.

Late-life depression is common but underrecognized and undertreated leading to significant morbidity and mortality, including from suicide. The presence of comorbidities necessitates screening followed by a careful history in order to make the diagnosis of depression. Because older adults tend to take longer to respond to treatment and have higher relapse rates than younger patients, they benefit most from persistent, attentive therapy. Although both pharmacotherapy and psychosocial treatments, or a combination of the two, are considered as the first-line therapy for late-life depression, most data support a combined, biopsychosocial treatment approach provided by an interdisciplinary team.

PRIMARY CARE:
CLINICS IN OFFICE PRACTICE

SERIES OF RELATED INTEREST

Medical Clinics (http://www.medical.theclinics.com)
Physician Assistant Clinics (https://www.physicianassistant.theclinics.com)

THE CLINICS ARE AVAILABLE ONLINE!
Access your subscription at:
www.theclinics.com

Dedications

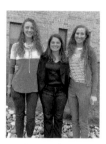

Erin Smith, DO;
Angela Colistra, PhD, LPC,
CAADC, CCS; and
Andrea Ward, DO

To all the people in training, the future rests in your hands. This fight for a more equitable SUD treatment landscape is one we will have to demand from systems and payers, but the fight is worth it because we do it for those we love.

Angela Colistra, Ph.D., LPC, CAADC, CCS: Growing up in West Virginia and starting my career in Appalachia, I saw the devastation of opioid addiction losing upwards to 20 friends and family members before I would reach my early 20s by the early 2000s. This reality moved me to further my education to help people heal and become trained to do addiction and mental health work. Far too many communities, families, and people continue to struggle with the devastation of addiction: access to evidenced-based care and affordability remains a challenge. To all those people who have lost their battle too early, I fight for a more equitable treatment landscape. To the 100s of people I have met along the way who have recovered, who are still fighting, and who have lost their battle, this work has always been for you and about you.

Andrea Ward, DO: To the people of eastern Kentucky who raised me in my early days of medicine, taught me through their needs, allowed me to listen to their stories, showed me their experiences with the plague of stigma, welcomed me with open arms, invited me to family dinners, and motivated me to become the best doctor I can be, my work in this was done for and with you held close in my heart. Thank you for exemplifying so astutely that the work of helping neighbors in need is what makes life worth living.

Erin Smith, DO: I dedicate this article *(Health Disparities, Substance Use Disorders, Primary Care)* to my mother, a strong and complex human being who struggled with addiction throughout her life and entered recovery in her early sixties. Thank you, mom, for showing us all that change is possible–for every one of us. Thank you for never giving up on yourself. Thank you for vulnerability, for trying again–and again–and again, and for showing us that while life is complicated, the light and dark come together and weave a quilt of our most precious gift of all: a full life.

Prim Care Clin Office Pract 50 (2023) xi
https://doi.org/10.1016/j.pop.2022.12.003
0095-4543/23/© 2022 Published by Elsevier Inc.

Foreword

We Are Here for You

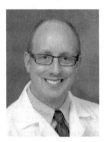

Joel J. Heidelbaugh, MD, FAAFP, FACG
Consulting Editor

"Thank you, thank you so much doctor for listening to me, for always being there for me. Even though I can't get to the office, just the ability to see you on video and have you listen to me for 15 minutes has brightened my day. I don't want to take medications; I just need someone to listen to what's been going on. I can't thank you enough. I have been so incredibly anxious and depressed lately. Don't worry, I'm not going to harm myself or anyone else. I just want to get some peace of mind. What do you think about using one of those cell phone apps to help my mood? Do they even work? Can we chat again next month? In the meantime, do you think staying off of social media will help my moods? Sometimes people can be so mean." (paraphrased, yet near verbatim)

Examples of similar patient encounters such as this one I experienced last week are exceedingly common in our practices. To say that "the world has changed" since the beginning of the COVID-19 pandemic in March 2020 is a vast understatement. Few would argue that people are less stressed, less anxious, or less depressed. Prior to the pandemic, there was a substantial and often unmet need for mental health services across our practices. Since 2020, the demand for these services has multiplied to the point of visible and crippling shortages that have created delays in care, greater utilization of urgent and emergent care services, and often the absence of care addressing the need for mental health support. I have been a family physician for over 23 years and still practice broad-spectrum primary care except obstetrics. While I am neither a psychiatrist nor a therapist, I often function in the role of one or both every single day in some capacity.

This issue of *Primary Care: Clinics in Office Practice* addresses many salient topics and concepts germane to addressing and managing the mental health needs of our patients in primary care practices. The issue commences with a stimulating article highlighting motivational interviewing skills, a concept rarely and inadequately taught in most medical education settings, and one which takes a significant length of time within one's career to come close to mastering. A novel concept for an article follows, one that dives deep into the utility of mobile apps for treating depression. Certainly, as mental health care resources have contracted and the demand for timely services has skyrocketed, alternative methods of care including self-help options have sprung to the forefront of patient-directed opportunity. Additional articles address the spectrum of attention-deficit disorder both with and without hyperactivity, disparities across patients with substance abuse disorders, suicide, adjustment disorders, eating disorders, obsessive-compulsive disorders, postpartum depression, and depression in the geriatric population. While I learned much new material and skills from each article, I likely learned the most from the article on adverse childhood events and trauma-informed care. This is a rapidly evolving area with great research that provides relevant awareness with the potential for shaping the care we deliver in a much more patient-centered fashion.

I would like to thank Dr Meagan Vermeulen, who did a superlative job as the guest editor of this issue in creating a practical and varied collection of articles centered on important topics in mental health issues we commonly encounter in primary care. I trust that this issue of *Primary Care: Clinics in Office Practice* will serve as a benchmark for both clinical practice and education across many levels. I would also like to acknowledge the many knowledgeable authors who provided detailed and well-written articles highlighting the current literature. Similar to our recent *Primary Care: Clinics in Office Practice* issues, it is my hope that this compendium will serve as an educational tool for students and residents across a wide variety of medical fields, as the information herein is applicable to nearly every specialty of health care. Most importantly to our patients, know that we are always here for you.

Joel J. Heidelbaugh, MD, FAAFP, FACG
Departments of Family Medicine and Urology
Department of Family Medicine
University of Michigan Medical School
Ann Arbor, MI 48109, USA

Ypsilanti Health Center
200 Arnet Suite 200
Ypsilanti, MI 48198, USA

E-mail address:
jheidel@umich.edu

Preface

Bridging the Gaps: Managing Behavioral Health in Primary Care

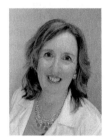

Meagan W. Vermeulen, MD, FAAFP
Editor

In its history, primary care has often been referred to as the "jack of all trades," with its purposefully broad base of training spanning the entire lifespan of our patients. This challenging field not only places us at the center of a patient's care team but also simultaneously creates and perpetuates the dynamic that is central to our identity as primary care providers: continuity of care. Primary care physicians not only routinely address a multitude of physical ailments but also are increasingly the first and only stop for patients on the winding, twisting path of identifying and caring for mental health disorders. Not only are the proper diagnosis and treatment of primary mental health disorders essential but also undiagnosed and improperly managed behavioral health conditions have the capacity to wreak havoc on the management of other chronic illnesses. If a patient truly isn't well emotionally, their ability to engage in a meaningful treatment plan for any other medical problem is limited at best, thus tying our hands further in the management of already complex individuals. In addition, despite decades of public education, the specter of stigma that cloaks most behavioral health diagnoses, let alone their treatment, is still very real for many of our patients. In addition, it is not uncommon that primary care providers shy away from managing these conditions. Whether it be a lack of formal training, a paucity of time and/or resources, or a general discomfort in managing behavioral health diagnoses, patients often feel lost in their attempts to engage in meaningful treatment plans for their behavioral health complaints. It's even more challenging for those whom a diagnosis is not straightforward or readily apparent, particularly if they inhabit any one of a multitude of marginalized identities. These vulnerable patients are often simply lost in the turbulent sea that is health care today with little hope of true recovery.

Despite these barriers, there is opportunity for hope. Our ability to develop lasting relationships by deploying expert communication skills while leaning on the essential

Prim Care Clin Office Pract 50 (2023) xv–xvi
https://doi.org/10.1016/j.pop.2022.11.007
0095-4543/23/© 2022 Published by Elsevier Inc.

skill to pivot can allow primary care physicians to succeed and thrive in our commitment to treating the whole person, *including* properly diagnosing and managing a multitude of behavioral health disorders. Because of the core tenets of our specialty: our wide-ranging breadth of expertise, the commitment to patient education, and the inherent longevity of our relationships with patients, primary care is uniquely positioned to light the way on this path too often filled with shadows.

Not only does this issue of *Primary Care: Clinics in Office Practice* represent a guide for the diagnosis and management of common behavioral health disorders in the primary care setting but it also represents a model for what the future of delivering care for behavioral health disorders could look like: a system of truly collaborative, integrated care. The authors in this issue cross multiple disciplines with expertise in a wide array of fields, including behavioral health, nutrition, addiction, and family medicine. What they all have in common is a dedication to putting the patient at the center of the care model while standing at a patient's side as advocates, educators, and guides on this journey through treating behavioral health in the primary care setting.

Meagan W. Vermeulen, MD, FAAFP
Department of Family Medicine
Rowan-Virtua School of Osteopathic Medicine
Sewell Campus: 1474 Tanyard Road Suite D100
Sewell, NJ 08080, USA

E-mail address:
vermeulen@rowan.edu

Motivational Interviewing in Primary-Care
Substance Use Disorders beyond AUDIT/DAST

Joanna Petrides, MBS, PsyD[a,b]

KEYWORDS

- Motivational interviewing • Substance-use • Primary-care • Mental health

KEY POINTS

- Primary-care physicians have a distinct opportunity to provide counseling regarding substance-use behaviors and to support patients in making behavioral changes.
- Motivational interviewing is a conversational style physicians can use to facilitate and support patients' desire for making behavioral changes.
- The spirit of motivational interviewing includes establishing a collaborative partnership between the patient and provider, evoking from patients what they care about as a conduit toward change, and honoring the patient's autonomy in decision making.
- The OARS approach is one interaction technique physicians can use in motivational interviewing and it includes the use of open-ended questions, affirmations, reflective listening, and summaries.
- Physicians should avoid engaging in certain traps when speaking with patients about creating behavioral changes such as arguing with resistance and the expert, labeling, and question–answer traps.

SUBSTANCE-USE DISORDERS IN THE PRIMARY-CARE SETTING
Prevalence of Substance-Use Disorders

Results from the 2020 National Survey on Drug Use and Health show 58.7% of people age 12 or older reported using substances including tobacco, alcohol, and illicit drugs within the past month,[1] with this rate likely higher in subsequent years as a result of the coronavirus disease-2019 (COVID-19) pandemic effects. Among the illicit substances, the most commonly used was marijuana, followed by stimulants (cocaine,

[a] Department of Family Medicine, Rowan-Virtua School of Osteopathic Medicine, 42 East Laurel Road, Suite 2100A, Stratford, NJ 08084, USA; [b] Department of Psychology, Rowan-Virtua School of Osteopathic Medicine, 42 East Laurel Road, Suite 2100A, Stratford, NJ 08084, USA
E-mail address: petrides@rowan.edu

Prim Care Clin Office Pract 50 (2023) 1–10
https://doi.org/10.1016/j.pop.2022.10.009   primarycare.theclinics.com

methamphetamine, and prescription stimulants), opioids (heroin or prescription pain relievers), non-opioid prescription pain relievers, and hallucinogens.[1]

Unfortunately, of those individuals age 12 or older needing substance-use treatment, only 1.4% received any kind of treatment in 2020.[1] The lack of engagement in substance-use treatment can be attributed to the limited access to specialized substance-use treatment programs and limitations brought on by the COVID-19 pandemic, among other reasons. Untreated and escalating patient substance-use behaviors not only affect the individual and their families, but also drive up the cost of health care.[2] With access to specialized substance-use treatment being limited, primary-care settings become a key site for addressing substance-use behaviors with patients, preventing substance-use from progressing into more problematic levels, and facilitating change in substance-use behaviors.

Use of Pre-Screening/Screening Tools in Primary-Care Settings

Addressing substance-use disorders has long been an element of patient care in the primary-care setting given that primary-care providers have established long-term relationships with their patients based on trust, and primary-care is considered a "gateway" to other specialties, often making it the patient's first stop in treating any chronic condition. A recent study confirmed screenings for substance-use in primary-care settings helped identify patients with problematic substance-use behaviors and those with multiple substance-use disorders.[3] Furthermore, awareness of patient substance-use in primary-care also assists in the effective treatment planning for problematic substance-use and other chronic conditions.[3]

The US Preventive Services Task Force (USPSTF) recommends screening all adults age 18 or older for unhealthy drug use by asking them questions about use and that screening should be conducted when services for accurate diagnosis, effective treatment, and appropriate care can be offered or referred.[4] The Substance Abuse and Mental Health Services Administration (SAMHSA) recommends the use of screening, brief intervention and referral to treatment (SBIRT) to assess severity of use and determine appropriate level of intervention.[5] SBIRT can be easily implemented into primary-care, emergency, and community settings to provide a comprehensive approach to screening and early intervention.[5] Screening is done with validated screening measures that show the severity of a patient's use. The most commonly used screening measures are the Alcohol-use Disorders Identification Test (AUDIT) for alcohol-use and the Drug Abuse Screen Test (DAST-10) for other substance-use.[6] Both measures are self-administered in the office setting, and reviewed and discussed with the health care provider. Screening for alcohol and substance-use are not limited to these measures and providers should use the screener that best fits their practice and patient needs.

Despite the effective implementation and use of screening tools in primary-care settings to identify the presence of substance-use problems, follow-up on addressing these problems has remained low, with lower follow-up rates occurring in rural areas.[7] A likely factor for this deficiency could be due to primary-care providers' limited understanding of approaches for and discomfort with engaging patients in conversations about substance-use practices. Beyond screening and providing patients with medical guidelines on recommended substance-use patterns for their health, many providers feel at a loss for how to engage their patients in discussing substance-use behavior and how to support them toward making a self-directed change. Motivational interviewing is a tool that provides physicians with a guide for having these difficult conversations successfully.

IMPLEMENTING MOTIVATIONAL INTERVIEWING FOR SUBSTANCE-USE INTO PRIMARY-CARE

Development of Motivational Interviewing

Motivational interviewing is a conversational style used toward fostering effective behavioral changes across a wide range of health behaviors.[8,9] Motivational interviewing was first developed in 1983 as a brief intervention for problematic alcohol-use and focused on addressing low levels of motivation as an obstacle to change.[8,9] Motivational interviewing has since been used and found effective with other health problems and chronic diseases in particular.[8,9] The mechanism of action for motivational interviewing is to elicit a patient's intrinsic motivation for making a behavioral change and adhere to treatment.[8,9]

Application of Motivational Interviewing

Conversations about changing behaviors develop organically and occur frequently in the primary-care setting, making it the ideal location for motivational interviewing to be incorporated. Motivational interviewing is a patient-centered approach focused on establishing a *collaborative* partnership between the patient and provider, *evoking* from the patient what they care about as a conduit toward change, and honoring the patient's *autonomy* in decision making.[8] This is knowns as the "spirit" of motivational interviewing.[8] Using this approach places the provider in a position of being a guide through change for patients by helping them develop an intrinsic motivation to change versus deciding the change path for the patient, which is typically ineffective.[10]

Using Motivational Interviewing to Move Change Along

Engaging in the process of developing change is a challenging undertaking for many people and this is especially true when making changes in substance-use behaviors. Patients with problematic substance-use behaviors often struggle with the ambivalence about making changes which is a factor in the continued use of substances. These patients can often be viewed as stuck, resistant, or unmotivated which leads providers to believe patients do not want to make changes.[9] Through the use of motivational interviewing, providers can identify this ambivalence to change and help transition it to meaningful action by using the patient's own motivating factors. It is important for the physician to be present in a nonjudgmental and open manner toward the patient to convey their support for the patient's process of making change. Some specific motivational interviewing techniques and approaches that are applicable in a primary-care setting will be discussed below.

RULE

Health care providers have a natural instinct to educate, persuade, and advise patients on necessary changes for improving their health.[9] However, it is human nature to resist persuasion from an outside source even in the face of unwanted health outcomes. Applying the guiding principles of motivational interviewing directs physicians away from pushing their own agenda onto the patient's change process.

There are four guiding principles of motivational interviewing and they are summarized using the acronym RULE, which stands for: resist the righting reflex (Resist), understand your patient's motivations (Understand), listen to your patient (Listen), and empower your patient (Empower).[8] Using the four guiding principles helps providers stay focused on what the patient is sharing and how this information can be used to direct the patient to make their self-defined changes (**Table 1**).

Table 1 RULE		
R	Resist the Righting Reflex	*Avoid telling, directing, or convincing the patient of the right path to good health*
U	Understand your Patient's Motivations	*Seek to understand your patient's perception of the situation and their motivation to change*
L	Listen to your Patient	*Seek to understand their values, needs, abilities, motivations, and potential barriers toward behavior changes*
E	Empower your Patient	*Support your patient's hope that change is possible and can make a difference in their health*

Data from Refs.[8,9]

Resisting the righting reflex is important for physicians to pay particular attention to. It can be difficult to resist guiding the patient to make a change that is important to their health; however, when being forceful with input about what changes the patient should make, the patient is likely to push against making this change. When physicians find themselves pushing for change while the patient resists, the provider is no longer in the role of a supporter toward change.[8] This emphasizes the importance for understanding what is behind the patient's interest in creating change. This self-identified motivation from the patient is something physicians can return to when the patient reaches a plateau or backslides in the change process to remind the patient their reason for change. To recognize this motivation, physicians should take the time to listen to the language from their patient, including listening for perceived barriers to change the patient identifies.[8] Lastly, the physician will act as a supportive partner for the patient through empowering the patient's ability to create change using the skills they already have and support their hope that such desired change is possible.[8]

Change Talk Versus Sustain Talk

The transtheoretical model of behavior change highlights the contemplative state of change as the point where patients are considering making a change but are not yet ready for change.[11] Patients who are not yet ready to make changes likely engage in sustain talk, which presents as language for why change is not possible.[12] Patients who use sustain talk are likely aware of the benefits in making changes and are also comfortable with their current status or there are disadvantages to making changes which they are not prepared to face.[12] Patients using sustain talk may say things similar to: "I know I need to change but I like the feeling I get from using drugs" or "I want to get sober but I'm afraid of the effects if I sober up." Motivational interviewing seeks to intervene at this stage. Within the scope of motivational interviewing, patients in the contemplative state experience ambivalence and physicians can assist patients in moving closer to change by listening for anything that indicates an openness or move toward change.[9] Sustain talk can shift to change talk through the use of reflections on the current behaviors, empathy for the patient's feelings, and recognizing that change is a personal choice of the patient.[9] Physicians can remember to listen for the different types of change talk using the acronym DARN-C (**Table 2**).

Table 2 DARN-C	
Desire	"I want to…" "I would like to…" "I wish…"
Ability	"I know I can…" "I am able to…" "I could…"
Reason	"I would probably feel better if I…" "My family would be happy if…" "I should do x because…"
Need	"Something has to change…" "I have to…" "I really should…"
Commitment	"I am going to…" "I will…" "I intend to…"

Data from Refs.[9,12]

OARS/EARS

Another approach of motivational interviewing which is used to engage the patient is using the microskills known as open questions, affirming, reflection and summarize (OARS).[9] Patients are often asked a series of close ended questions by health care providers, which either produce little information about what is actually going on or the patients are able to figure out which answer their provider prefers and answer in a way so as to satisfy their provider. This approach to question asking does little to help patients who are hesitant to bring up their substance-use and physicians are none the wiser about what the patient is struggling with. By asking open questions, patients are able to respond in their own way and it removes the physician from the "expert role," making it more comfortable for the patient and provider to engage in dialogue about change.[9] This also assists with building trust and acceptance.[9] Open questions are followed by affirming the patient's strengths and abilities.[9] Even small changes should be affirmed and physicians should avoid focusing on pathology or criticizing any limitations in achieving bigger changes. Physicians should use reflection to communicate empathy to patients.[9] This can be done by repeating part of what the patient said and using the patient's own words. Reflective listening solidifies that the physician understands the way the patient experiences the situation.[9] The last microskill physicians can use is to summarize, which lets the patient know their provider was listening and values what the patient shared.[9] Summaries are typically no longer than 3 or 4 sentences and are a good way to check in that both the patient and provider are on the same page.[9] An effective summary is able to link material together and emphasize significant points.[9]

Additionally, physicians can respond to a patient's change talk using elaborate/example, affirming, reflection, and summarize (EARS) to further elicit more change talk.[9] EARS is similar to OARS but focuses the questions on seeking more elaboration or an example to encourage the patient to continue exploring change talk.[9] These types of questions should be asked with curiosity and the objective is to better understand what the patient means by their change talk[9] **(Table 3)**.

Table 3 OARS/EARS			
O	Open Questions "How does this behavior affect you?" "How would you like things to be different?"	E	Elaborate/Example "In what ways do you think you would feel better?" "Give me an example of…"
A	Affirming "It took courage to do that" "That's a really good idea"	A	Affirming "Good for you!" "You really want to stay healthy."
R	Reflection "You're feeling ____ because ____." "It sounds like you…"	R	Reflection "You'd like to be making more progress."
S	Summarize "Let's go over what we talked about today." "Here is what I've heard. Tell me if I've missed anything."	S	Summarize "So far you have shared how your substance-use affects your relationships."

Data from Arkowitz H, Miller WR, Rollnick S, Miller WR, Arkowitz H. Learning, Applying and Extending Motivational Interviewing. In: Motivational Interviewing in the Treatment of Psychological Problems. New York, NY: The Guilford Press; 2017:1-32.

TRAPS TO AVOID

It is important to remember that motivational interviewing is a particular way of communicating and offering advice when appropriate. This is likely a different approach from the usual way physicians are accustomed to communicating with patients. As a result, there can be times where the physicians fall into traps of communicating in ineffective ways. A few common traps will be identified and explored below.

Expert Trap

Physicians are known and regarded as experts in their field of practice. It is therefore very natural to tell the patient what the physician thinks they should do when the patient asks something like "what should I do?" They would not be asking if they did not want their physician to given them a direction to follow, right? This approach is typically ineffective because patients rarely follow directions even if they know it is in their best interest. In the scope of motivational interviewing, advice is given in a specific way and with permission. Physicians are encouraged to hold back the urge of directly giving advice and instead to ask permission first. This can be done by saying something like "Would it be helpful if I shared with you some things other people have done and had success with?"[9] Following any advice given, the physician can follow-up with another question such as "Is this something that you would find helpful?"[9] This is known as the ask-provide-ask method and the aim of this approach is to emphasize the collaboration between patient and provider.[9,10]

Arguing with Resistance

When patients struggle with starting or progressing with change we can be quick to label the patient as resistant. It is easy to place the blame on the patient and imply it is a problem that is wholly theirs.[9] The current model of motivational interviewing has shifted away from focusing on resistance[10] after recognizing that much of the resistance was the presence of sustain talk stemming from the sense of ambivalence.[9] Furthermore, evidence supports that resistance is also a result of the patient

Table 4
Traps to Avoid

Trap	What It Looks like	What Is Should Look like
Expert trap	"Your level of use warrants admission to a rehabilitation center."	"Other patients have sought out treatment. Does this sound like something you'd like to try?"
Arguing with resistance	"You're not engaging with your treatment like you should be."	"I know these changes are big steps for you and they don't' always go as planned."
Labeling trap	"You are an alcoholic."	"How has your alcohol-use affected you?"
Question–answer trap	"Do you think you drink too much?"	"Tell me about your drinking pattern."

Data from Miller WR, Rollnick S. Motivational Interviewing: Helping People Change. New York, NY: Guilford Press; 2013.

responding to the provider's style[13,14] thus indicating that resistance is not one-sided and it is important to work together with the patient to move past resistance. Engaging with the resistance often involves the use of the word "you," such as "I'm not sure you can help me" or "You don't understand how hard this is."[9] These statements show the patient is feeling isolated rather than supported and is pushing back on the challenges of change. More automatic responses from the physician might be to explain to the patient how the provider can help them or tell them you understand what they are going through. Rolling with the resistance is a more efficient and effective approach. It involves using statements such as, "I understand this change is a big challenge for you and you're giving it your best effort" or "It sounds like you really want to get sober and you don't feel like other people understand how hard you're working on this change." When rolling with the resistance it shows empathy to the patient's efforts and collaboration in the process.[9]

Labeling Trap

Using labels in medicine is a commonly used way to communicate more in-depth information in a quick, condensed manner. However, applying a label such as "alcoholic," "drug user," or "resistant" to a patient makes them feel attacked and they become defensive.[10] This furthers the patient's resistance as they are responding to feeling as though their physician only sees them as a label and this can create a power struggle. Labels also do not take individual factors into consideration and are therefore ineffective in addressing what the patient is really dealing with. Instead of using a label to describe an issue, it is helpful to focus on how the issue is impacting the patient, such as what does the issue mean to the patient and how is it impacting the patient's ability to make progress.[10]

Question–Answer Trap

When physicians are in search of information about their patient, it can become easy to ask a series of close-ended questions that pull for a limited kind of response. This pattern of asking questions encourages the patient to provide short, simple answers that do not serve the purpose of robust information seeking. The question–answer trap also sets up the dynamic of the physician being the expert and the patient being a passive participant in the change process.[10] Lastly, this trap offers limited opportunities for the patient to share their own motivations and talk about change. Physicians

Table 5		
Additional Applications of Motivational Interviewing		
Diabetes	Major Depressive Disorder	Anxiety Disorders
Smoking cessation	Weight management	Asthma
Treatment adherence	Medication compliance	Improved quality of life

Data from Refs.[15,16]

can stay away from a question–answer trap through the use of open-ended questions that pull for more information and the patient's reflection on the issue[10] (**Table 4**).

HOW DOES MOTIVATIONAL INTERVIEWING FIT INTO A PRIMARY-CARE PRACTICE

As stated above, motivational interviewing is a patient-centered conversational style that can be applied to strengthen the patient-provider relationship and support the process of the patient's behavioral change. It is a helpful skill for all health care providers to have in their toolbox; however, schedule limitations can often hinder the physician's ability to apply this tool during a regular office visit. An alternative model of implementing motivational interviewing into a primary-care setting is through the use of allied health professionals such as health educators or recovery coaches.[2] Health educators and recovery coaches are trained in administering appropriate screening tools for assessing the severity of the issue, reviewing these results with patients in a manner that helps the patient understand the results of the assessment, and to begin the process of motivational interviewing with the aim of identifying the patient's readiness for change and partnering with the patient to identify change goals. Using a health educator or recovery coach provides both the patient and the physician additional support in initiating and maintaining changes. By having the health educator or recovery coach begin the change process, the physician can then check in with the patient's progress at a follow-up visit and use motivational interviewing to address progress, resistance, and/or plateauing.

USE OF MOTIVATIONAL INTERVIEWING IN PRIMARY-CARE BEYOND SUBSTANCE-USE DISORDERS

Since its development, motivational interviewing has been empirically validated for use with many chronic conditions that present in primary-care settings.[15,16] Some of the most common applications for motivational interviewing are included below. Physicians can apply the same conversational approaches and skills shared above to guide the patient from a place of being ambivalent to a place of making changes in service of their health (**Table 5**).

SUMMARY

Given the significant rate of substance-use behaviors among individuals age 12 or older in the United States,[1] which has likely worsened as a result of the COVID-19 pandemic effects, and the extremely low rate of substance-use treatment,[1] it is important for primary-care practices to recognize the important role they have in helping screen patients for substance-use behaviors and support them in guiding behavioral changes. Primary-care offices are accessed more easily and frequently by patients which allows for the ability to screen a high number of patients for substance-use and provide a brief intervention based on the patient's readiness for change.

Through the use of screening tools such as the AUDIT (for alcohol-use) and DAST (for drug use), primary-care providers can quickly and easily assess substance-use severity and frequency. Physicians can review these screening tools and begin supporting the patient's path to change using motivational interviewing techniques. By partnering with the patient to cultivate their intrinsic motivation, providers can move their patients from a place of ambivalence to making real change in service of their health. Several motivational interviewing techniques and examples were provided throughout this article.

Motivational interviewing is not limited to being used only to address substance-use behaviors. Motivational interviewing has been empirically validated for use with a wide range of chronic health care issues. Physicians can enlist the help of health educators and other allied health care providers in working with the patient in the primary-care setting toward developing and maintaining meaningful behavioral change.

CLINICS CARE POINTS

- The 2020 National Survey on Drug Use and Health showed 58.7% of people age 12 or older reported substance-use including tobacco, alcohol, and illicit drugs; however, only 1.4% received any kind of substance-use treatment in 2020.

- The primary-care setting is ripe for engaging in motivational interviewing, the patient-centered conversational approach, to address a multitude of health-focused behavioral changes, including substance-use, because of its ability to reach a wider net of patients.

- Motivational interviewing was first developed to address problematic alcohol-use and focused on addressing motivation as an obstacle to change.[8,9]

- Motivational interviewing aims to create a collaborative partnership between the patient and provider to evoke what the patient cares about all while honoring the patient's autonomy.

- Motivational interviewing skills include:
  - *RULE:* Resist the righting reflex; Understand your patient's motivations; Listen to your patient; and Empower your patient
  - *DARN-C:* Desire, Ability, Reason, Need, and Commitment
  - *OARS:* Open questions, Affirming, Reflection, Summarize
  - *EARS:* Elaborate/Example, Affirming, Reflection, Summarize

- Some of the traps to avoid when conducting motivational interviewing are:
  - Expert Trap
  - Arguing with Resistance
  - Labeling Trap
  - Question–answer Trap

- Motivational interviewing can be incorporated into primary-care settings with the help of a health educator or recovery coach who can facilitate the patient screening for problematic health behaviors, assess patient readiness for change, and use the conversational techniques to support the patient's change process.

DISCLOSURE

The author reports no financial conflict of interests.

REFERENCES

1. Substance Abuse and Mental Health Services Administration (SAMHSA). National Survey on Drug Use and Health (NSDUH) Annual National Report.

SAMHSA.gov. 2020. Available at: https://www.samhsa.gov/data/report/2020-nsduh-annual-national-report. Accessed April 12, 2022.

2. Jack HE, Oller D, Kelly J, et al. Addressing substance use disorder in primary-care: The role, integration, and impact of recovery coaches. Substance Abuse 2017;39(3):307–14. https://doi.org/10.1080/08897077.2017.1389802.

3. John WS, Zhu H, Mannelli P, et al. Prevalence, patterns, and correlates of multiple substance-use disorders among adult primary-care patients. Drug and Alcohol Dependence 2018;187:79–87. https://doi.org/10.1016/j.drugalcdep.2018.01.035.

4. Unhealthy drug use: Screening. Recommendation: Unhealthy Drug Use: Screening | United States Preventive Services Taskforce. 2020. Available at: https://www.uspreventiveservicestaskforce.org/uspstf/recommendation/drug-use-illicit-screening#:~:text=Recommendation%20Summary&text=The%20USPSTF%20recommends%20screening%20by,can%20be%20offered%20or%20referred. Accessed April 13, 2022.

5. About screening, brief intervention, and referral to treatment (SBIRT). SAMHSA. Available at: https://www.samhsa.gov/sbirt/about. Accessed April 13, 2022.

6. University of Missouri-Kansas City School of Nursing and Health Studies. Tools. Clinician Tools - SBIRT for Substance Abuse. Available at: https://www.sbirt.care/tools.aspx. Accessed April 13, 2022.

7. Chan YF, Lu SE, Howe B, et al. Screening and Follow-Up Monitoring for Substance-use in Primary-care: An Exploration of Rural–Urban Variations. J GEN INTERN MED 2016;31:215–22. https://doi.org/10.1007/s11606-015-3488-y.

8. Rollnick S, Miller WR, Butler C. Motivational Interviewing: Principles and Evidence. In: Motivational interviewing in health care: helping patients change behavior. New York, NY: The Guilford Press; 2022. p. 3–10.

9. Arkowitz H, Miller WR, Rollnick S, et al. Learning, Applying and Extending Motivational Interviewing. In: Motivational interviewing in the treatment of Psychological problems. New York, NY: The Guilford Press; 2017. p. 1–32.

10. Miller WR, Rollnick S. Motivational interviewing: helping people change. New York, NY: Guilford Press; 2013.

11. Prochaska JO, DiClemente CC. Transtheoretical therapy: Toward a more integrative model of change. Psychotherapy: Theor Res Pract 1982;19(3):276–88.

12. Rollnick S, Miller WR, Butler C. Practicing Motivational Interviewing. In: Motivational interviewing in health care: helping patients change behavior. New York, NY: The Guilford Press; 2022. p. 33–43.

13. Glynn LH, Moyers TB. Chasing change talk: The Clinician's role in evoking client language about change. J Substance Abuse Treat 2010;39(1):65–70.

14. Patterson GR, Forgatch MS. Therapist behavior as a determinant for client noncompliance: A paradox for the behavior modifier. J Consulting Clin Psychol 1985;53(6):846–51.

15. Lundahl B, Moleni T, Burke BL, et al. Motivational interviewing in Medical Care Settings: A systematic review and meta-analysis of randomized controlled trials. Patient Education Couns 2013;93(2):157–68.

16. Britt E, Hudson SM, Blampied NM. Motivational interviewing in Health Settings: A Review. Patient Education Couns 2004;53(2):147–55.

Use of Mobile Apps & Stepped-Care Model for Treating Depression in Primary Care

Krista L. Herbert, PhD[a],*, James Michael M. Brennan, PhD[b]

KEYWORDS

- Stepped-care • Depression • Primary care • Mobile apps
- Measurement-based care

KEY POINTS

- Measurement-based care is used to assess severity of a patient's symptoms and interventions are prescribed that match the severity of symptoms and patient preferences.
- Stepped-care has 2 key principles that are critical to consider when treatment planning: (1) symptoms are continually monitored and patients can step up or down in levels of treatment depending on their clinical response to an intervention and (2) neither the cost nor the intensity of an intervention is related to its effectiveness.
- Therefore, a variety of evidence-based treatment options are available for patients, including watchful waiting, psychoeducation and/or self-help (eg, bibliotherapy, mobile apps), pharmacotherapy and/or psychotherapy, and intensive outpatient or inpatient services.

INTRODUCTION

Primary care has become the first and only point of contact for a majority of individuals experiencing psychological problems, with estimates showing that 40% to 70% of primary care visits are focused on mental health-related concerns.[1,2] Of the psychological services accessed in primary care, depression-related symptoms are a major driver.[3,4] Although the standard of care for treating depression within primary care typically involves prescribing antidepressant medication, referral for outpatient psychotherapy, or some combination of these 2 treatments, many patients do not follow through with these recommendations.[5,6] For example, it is estimated that 50% to 90% of patients do not follow through with mental health referrals and for

[a] VA Portland Health Care System, 3710 Southwest US Veterans Hospital Road, Portland, OR 97239, USA; [b] San Francisco VA Health Care System, 4150 Clement Street, San Francisco, CA 94121, USA
* Corresponding author.
E-mail address: Krista.Herbert@va.gov

Prim Care Clin Office Pract 50 (2023) 11–19
https://doi.org/10.1016/j.pop.2022.10.005
0095-4543/23/Published by Elsevier Inc.

those who do initiate mental health care, coordination and collaboration of care between the primary care physician and mental health professionals are rare.[2] Considering the obstacles of treating depression within primary care, alternative models of care have been developed to address problems with access, effectiveness, and efficiency, as well as patient and provider satisfaction of mental health treatment within primary care.

Stepped-Care Models

In recent years, stepped-care (SC) models have been adopted in primary care settings as an alternative to standard care for people endorsing psychological concerns. Treatment decisions within the SC model are influenced by assessment, evidence-based practice, and collaboration with the patient to determine potential treatment preferences and appropriate interventions.[7] Additionally, SC models aim to provide the least intensive, yet most effective intervention as the first step of care for all patients.[8] Progression in treatment is monitored on a weekly basis and patients are stepped up or down in level of care depending on their clinical response to the intervention. As a result, SC offers a variety of interventions that range from low to high intensity (eg, from watchful waiting to intensive outpatient mental health services).[7,9]

In order to implement SC, individuals experiencing mental health symptoms must be identified in a timely manner and symptom severity must be assessed. Therefore, this model requires implementation of routine screening and assessment of mental health symptoms with a primary care setting as part of a larger clinic-wide screening program or triggered by patient self-report.[7,9] Screening instruments that have been validated for their population and setting (ie, primary care) include the Patient Health Questionnaire (PHQ-9) and the Generalized Anxiety Disorder-7 scales (GAD-7). Implementation of screening has not only led to increased rates of identifying patients experiencing depressive symptoms but when paired with an intervention, individuals are more likely to experience a greater reduction of symptoms and response to interventions.[10,11]

Once patients are identified, SC mandates that their preferences be considered as part of a collaborative process of decision-making and treatment planning.[9] This framework comes from the psychotherapy outcomes studies, which suggest that incorporating the patient's treatment preference throughout treatment improves clinical outcome,[12] adherence[13] and reduces rates of attrition.[14] Based on the severity of symptoms, providers present patients with a variety of the interventions clinically indicated for the level of symptomology. For example, if a patient endorsed a score of 16 on the PHQ-9, which is indicative of moderately severe depressive symptoms, a provider may recommend psychotherapy and/or medication. Ongoing monitoring of symptoms through measurement-based care will help provider's determine if and when a patient should be stepped-up to a higher level of care.

Treatments Offered Within Each Step

Step 1: *Watchful Waiting*. Watchful waiting is a nondirective approach to care and involves initial screening and identification of mental health symptoms, education on warning signs of increasing symptomology, and weekly monitoring of symptoms. Although watchful waiting is not an active treatment, there is evidence to suggest that certain mental health conditions, such as depression and anxiety, naturally remit over time and resolve without intervention.[7,9] For example, Patten and colleagues[15] found that 16% of individuals diagnosed with a mild episode of major depressive disorder receiving watchful waiting recovered within 2 weeks of the initial diagnosis, and an additional 30% recovered in 4 weeks. Considering these data, watchful waiting is recommended for individuals:

- Experiencing minimal to mild levels of depressive symptoms (eg, scores between 1 and 9 on the PHQ-9),
- Whose symptoms do not interfere with daily functioning or cause notable distress,
- Whose symptoms are a result of an acute stress that is expected to be resolved in a short period of time,
- Have no previous mental health history,
- Deny current and historical suicidal ideation, and
- Prefer or are willing to wait a few weeks to see if symptoms remit.

Although this intervention may be effective for patients meeting the criteria above, it is not recommended for those experiencing panic symptoms,[16] posttraumatic stress disorder,[17] or social anxiety disorder[18] because these disorders tend to be chronic and show very low rates of spontaneous remission. Regarding alcohol and substance use, watchful waiting should only be recommended for individuals experiencing sub-threshold symptoms of an alcohol or substance use disorder because there is some evidence to suggest that self-monitoring alone can reduce alcohol and substance use.[19]

Depending on the specific symptoms and precipitating factors, it is possible that some patients may actually prefer watchful waiting over an active treatment. For example, Dwight and colleagues[20] found that patients who preferred watchful waiting were more likely to have less knowledge about depression because of first experience of depressive symptoms.

It is recommended that the patient's symptoms are monitored during the course of 4 weeks because improvements or worsening of symptoms usually occur within this time frame.[7,15] During this time, patients would be encouraged to complete self-report measures at least once per week. With increased efforts to improve screening and advancements in technology, patients can easily access measures (eg, PHQ-9 and GAD-7) online. If symptoms persist or increase in severity, they would be encouraged to return to the primary care office to discuss further stepped-up treatment options.

Step 2: *Psychoeducation and/or self-help interventions.* In the event that watchful waiting does not result in the remittance of symptoms or leads to an increase in acuity, providers and patients should consider a stepped-up intervention. These are described below.

Psychoeducation. Although psychoeducation is the pillar of all psychotherapeutic interventions, empirical evidence suggests that psychoeducation alone can be effective for treating mild levels of symptoms of anxiety and depression.[7,9] This intervention can include providing information on the nature and course of disorders, bio-psychosocial factors that cause and maintain symptomology, and various treatment options (eg, exercise, therapy, medications).[9] Information can be delivered through websites, videos, pamphlets, books, mobile apps, and classes/groups.

Self-help interventions. Self-help interventions offer skills and techniques for individuals to manage symptoms on their own and implement behavioral change.[7] Self-help interventions include bibliotherapy, Internet-based interventions, and mobile applications (apps). Self-help interventions can be guided or unguided. Unguided self-help interventions do not include any assistance from a mental health professional and can be completed fully on one's own. Conversely, guided self-help consists of mental health professionals providing instructions regarding how to best use self-help interventions (eg, frequency of engagement and review of skills/tools/features), answering questions about navigating the intervention, and assessing progress and needs. Research examining the effectiveness of guided versus unguided self-help interventions suggests that guided self-help interventions are more effective than unguided interventions.[21,22]

It is vital that the primary care provider and/or mental health professional familiarize themselves with the specific self-help intervention before recommending it to a patient in order to more effectively support their utilization of this intervention. Frequency of contact may vary pending the type of intervention selected, the patient's comfort level, and severity of symptomology. However, independent of these factors, increased contact with a member of their health-care team may serve as a reminder to engage with the self-help material and increase adherence. Moreover, conducting weekly or biweekly checks in with patients using self-help will provide an opportunity not only to assess their progress with and utilization of the intervention but also to complete or review assessment measures in order to determine whether stepping up to a higher level of care is necessary. As with watchful waiting, if symptoms persist or increase in severity over the course of 1 month, patients would be encouraged to step-up to the next level of care.

A majority of self-help interventions include evidenced-based practices, such as cognitive-behavioral therapy, problem-solving therapy, behavioral activation (BA), mindfulness, and acceptance and commitment approaches.[7] Self-help interventions are not only cost-effective but have been found to be comparable to traditional psychotherapy for treating mild to moderate levels of depression and anxiety (eg, those endorsing scores between 5 and 14 on the PHQ-9).[11,23–25] In addition, self-help interventions may be most effective for individuals who:

- Deny current suicidal ideation,
- Endorse a preference for self-help,
- Report higher levels of motivation and confidence in their ability to make behavioral changes on their own,
- Have access to reliable Internet services and own a smartphone or computer, and
- Experience numerous barriers accessing and engaging in psychotherapy services (eg, transportation issues, financial concerns, community waitlists for treatment).

mHealth. Using mobile apps as a delivery system for self-help interventions has received considerable attention by researchers, providers, and the public. Mobile apps have distinct advantages over traditional mental health interventions, including lower costs, increased treatment accessibility, and greater retention.[26] Further, mobile apps provide individuals with the opportunity to track and monitor their symptoms and progress in real-time, which is a more accurate representation of their experience of symptoms and influence on daily life. Thus, if individuals can monitor and track their symptoms and progress, they may be more inclined to adhere to the recommended treatment.[27]

Preliminary evidence suggests that using mobile apps can reduce depressive symptoms. For example, in their meta-analysis of 18 randomized controlled trials with 22 mobile apps, Firth and colleagues[28] found that individuals using mobile apps to manage depressive symptoms experienced a significant reduction of symptoms when compared with control conditions ($g = 0.38$, $P < .001$). The authors reported moderate effect sizes compared with inactive control groups ($g = 0.56$) and small effect sizes compared with an active control condition ($g = 0.22$).

However, it is important to note that most apps currently available to the general public have been inadequately evaluated for their effectiveness in treating depressive symptoms.[26,28] For example, Martinez-Perez and colleagues[29] found that out of 1536 depression apps available in app stores, only 32 published articles evaluated the effectiveness of depression apps. Additionally, there are concerns regarding the consistency between mobile apps and evidence-based therapy practices. In their systematic review of 117 depression mobile apps that purported to offer cognitive behavioral therapy (CBT) or BA, Huguet and colleagues[30] found that only 12 of those apps were consistent with the theories and principles of CBT and BA.

Given the heterogeneity of the apps available, it is key that providers help patients select the most appropriate app for their needs. Additionally, the use of mobile apps allows for greater flexibility and inclusion of patient preference given the vast amount of apps that have been developed based on the different theoretical orientations. Thus, a provider could recommend a mobile app that aligns with the patient's preferred theoretical orientation. To assist with this endeavor, the American Psychological Association's Society for Clinical Psychology, Anxiety and Depression Association of America, and One Mind PsyberGuide have published guides of mobile apps that are empirically support or evaluated by mental health professionals for consistency with evidence-based practices. Additionally, the US Department of Veterans Affairs has developed and researched mobile apps for a multiple of diagnoses that are not only consistent with evidence-based practices but also free to download for iPhone and Android users.

Step 3: *Psychotherapy and/or Psychotropic Medication*. After careful monitoring of patient responses to treatment in steps 1 and 2, more traditional and comprehensive mental health treatment may be indicated. This could include individual or group psychotherapy, and/or psychotropic medication, depending on patient interest and preferences. It would also be consistent with the SC model to initiate step 3 interventions from the outset if individuals are experiencing moderate-to-severe symptoms (ie, endorse scores of 10 or higher on the PHQ-9), have a strong preference for psychotherapy and/or medications, report higher levels of impairment in functioning, and endorse suicidal ideations.[7,9] Based on current treatment guidelines, individuals experiencing moderate symptoms of depression may benefit from psychotherapy or medication alone, whereas those endorsing severe symptomology may experience the greatest reduction of symptoms when using a combination of psychotherapy and medication.[8]

Step 4: *Intensive Outpatient, Partial Day Programs, or Inpatient Care*. Intensive outpatient, partial day, and inpatient care is considered the most intensive level of care. Individuals at this level of care would be referred to a specialty mental health facility. Intensive outpatient and partial day programs may be most effective for individual who:

- Endorse severe depressive symptoms (ie, 19 or higher on the PHQ-9),
- Have suicidal and/or homicidal ideation,
- Have a stable and supportive living environment,
- Have access to and agree to utilize a safety plan, and
- are agreeable to a follow-up plan.

The goal of inpatient services is to stabilize individuals experiencing severe depressed symptoms and active suicidal and homicidal ideation.[7] Intensive outpatient or partial day programs include actively attending a program 3 to 5 times a week that can last anywhere from 3 to 6 hours each day. During this time, the patient would engage in individual and group psychotherapy services. On discharge from these services, interventions from the 3 other steps may be warranted to support patients in their recovery.

Empirical Evidence

The SC model offers benefits based on access, patient engagement, and practicability for providers and interdisciplinary health-care teams. Assessment of the effectiveness of this model remains mixed and its greatest strength may be is acceptability to patients. For example, Seekles and colleagues[31] examined the effectiveness of the SC model for primary care patients with anxiety and depressive symptoms. Results indicated that there were no significant differences between patients in the SC or standard of care conditions on either depression or anxious symptoms at the 8-week, 16-week, or 24-week follow-ups. Additionally, van Straten and colleagues[32] found limited evidence to support the notion that the SC is more effective than standard of care. However, in their meta-analytic review, Firth and colleagues[12] found small-to-moderate effect sizes in favor of the SC model when compared with standard of care. Given the magnitude of the mental health need, even small improvements can make a big cumulative impact.

Importantly, these authors found that patient acceptability of treatment moderated the overall effectiveness of the SC model, with those studies reporting a significantly greater satisfaction with the SC model having greater overall clinical outcome when compared with standard of care. Regarding the cost-effectiveness of the SC, the data are inconsistent. To date, only 2 studies have examined the difference in costs between SC and standard of care, with one study reporting no significant differences in total mean cost of treatment,[33] whereas the other reported that the SC model reduced costs and incidence rates of depression by approximately 50%.[34]

DISCUSSION

Increasingly, primary care is the first line of intervention for mental health concerns, yet existing standards of care have not been sufficient to address the need. SC models provide an alternative approach that is targeted and algorithmic, easily adaptable, and closely aligned with patient preferences. Using validated mental health screeners, providers can recommend interventions targeted to the needs of the patient with the option to step up or step down care as indicated. Having such a model creates usability for providers through clear decision-making procedures and identified treatment modalities and clear next steps based on outcomes. SC models benefit from patient input and collaboration around assessment, treatment choice, and step changes. This orientation not only increases trust and transparency but also contributes to improved adherence and clinical outcomes.

The SC model makes treatment available for patients with a wide-range of symptom presentations and can adjust to fluctuations in symptom severity longitudinally. Step 1 targets mild symptoms and focuses on watchful waiting, which increases patient awareness of symptoms, accounts for the psychological consequences of common life stressors, allows for the natural remittance of mild symptoms, and establishes a clear baseline for symptoms to inform follow-up. Step 2 targets mild and moderate symptoms that have not remitted or have increased in severity. This step uses psychoeducation, self-help interventions, and mobile health options that provide patients with highly accessible and empirically based interventions. Steps 1 and 2 recognize the potency of empirically based, low-cost treatments. Steps 3 and 4 provide options for heightened care for those requiring a higher level of care and include psychopharmacological intervention, psychotherapy, and intensive outpatient and inpatient care.

SUMMARY

The SC model of care is an innovative framework for targeting mental health needs in the primary care setting. Its advantages include assisting patients and their interdisciplinary teams make decisions regarding care as well as optimizing the broad range of mental health services currently available, including self-help and mobile interventions. The SC model offers a patient-centered, provider-friendly, and potentially cost-effective approach to managing primary care patients mental health needs.

CLINICS CARE POINTS

- Patients should be monitored on a weekly basis and can be stepped up to a higher level of care if symptoms increase in severity after 1 month.
- The cost and intensity of an intervention are not related to its effectiveness. As a result, patients experiencing mild-to-moderate symptoms of depression can begin with an evidence-based treatment of low cost and intensity, such as bibliotherapy or mobile apps.
- Providers should be flexible with treatment recommendations and consider patient preferences and needs, and systemic barriers to accessing care when creating treatment plans.

DISCLOSURE

The authors K L. Herbert and J M M. Brennan declare that they have no conflict of interest.

ACKNOWLEDGMENTS

The authors would like to thank the editors for the opportunity to contribute to this publication.

REFERENCES

1. Hunter CL, Goodie JL, Oordt MS, et al. Introduction. In: Integrated behavioral health in primary care: Step-by-Step guidance for assessment and intervention. 2nd edition. American Psychological Association; 2017. p. 3–8. https://doi.org/10.1037/0000017-001.
2. Kessler R, Stafford D. Primary Care Is the De Facto Mental Health System. In: Kessler R, Stafford D, editors. Collaborative medicine case Studies: evidence in practice. New York: Springer Science & Business Media; 2008. p. 1–440.
3. Mitchell AJ, Vaze A, Rao S. Clinical diagnosis of depression in primary care: a meta-analysis. Lancet 2009;374(9690):609–19.
4. Pignone MP, Gaynes BN, Rushton JL, et al. Screening for Depression in Adults: A Summary of the Evidence for the U.S. Preventive Services Task Force. Ann Intern Med 2002;136(10):765.
5. Trangle M, Gursky J, Haight R, Hardwig J, Hinnenkamp T, Kessler D, Mack N, Myszkowski M. Institute for Clinical Systems Improvement. Adult Depression in Primary Care. Updated March 2016. Available at: Depr.pdf (icsi.org)
6. Sansone RA, Sansone LA. Antidepressant Adherence: Are Patients Taking Their Medications? Innov Clin Neurosci 2012;9(4–5):41–6.

7. Broten LA, Naugle AE, Kalata AH, et al. Depression and a Stepped Care Model. In: O'Donohue WT, Draper C, editors. Stepped care and E-health: practical applications to behavioral disorders. New york: Spring; 2011. p. 1–328.

8. National Institute for Health and Clinical Excellence. Depression: Evidence Update April 2012. 2012. https://www.nice.org.uk/guidance/cg90/evidence/evidence-update-pdf-243829405. [Accessed 24 April 2022].

9. O'Donohue WT, Draper C. The case for evidence-based stepped care as part of a reformed delivery system. In: O'Donohue WT, Draper C, editors. Stepped care and E-health: practical applications to behavioral disorders. New York: Spring; 2011. p. 1–328.

10. O'Connor E, Rossom RC, Henninger M, et al. Screening for Depression in Adults: An Updated Systematic Evidence Review for the U.S. Preventive Services Task Force. Agency for Healthcare Research and Quality (US), Rockville (MD); 2016. PMID: 26937538.

11. Smithson S, Pignone MP. Screening Adults for Depression in Primary Care. Med Clin North Am 2017;101(4):807–21.

12. Firth N, Barkham M, Kellett S. The clinical effectiveness of stepped care systems for depression in working age adults: A systematic review. J Affect Disord 2015; 170:119–30.

13. Kwan BM, Dimidjian S, Rizvi SL. Treatment preference, engagement, and clinical improvement in pharmacotherapy versus psychotherapy for depression. Behav Res Ther 2010;48(8):799–804.

14. Swift JK, Greenberg RP. Incorporate preferences into the treatment decision-making process. In: Premature termination in psychotherapy: strategies for engaging clients and improving outcomes. American Psychological Association; 2015. p. 79–92. https://doi.org/10.1037/14469-007.

15. Patten SB, Williams JVA, Lavorato DH, et al. Major depression as a risk factor for chronic disease incidence: longitudinal analyses in a general population cohort. Gen Hosp Psychiatry 2008;30(5):407–13.

16. Andersson G, Carlbring P. Panic Disorder. In: O'Donohue WT, Draper C, editors. Stepped care and E-health: practical applications to behavioral disorders. New York: Spring; 2011. p. 1–328.

17. Draper C, Ghiglieri M. Post-traumatic Stress Disorder: Computer-Based Stepped Care: Practical Applications to Clinical Problems. In: O'Donohue WT, Draper C, editors. Stepped care and E-health: practical applications to behavioral disorders. New York: Spring; 2011. p. 1–328.

18. Andersson G, Carlbring P. Social Phobia (Social Anxiety Disorder). In: O'Donohue WT, Draper C, editors. Stepped care and E-health: practical applications to behavioral disorders. New York: Spring; 2011. p. 1–328.

19. Clifford PR, Maisto SA. Subject reactivity effects and alcohol treatment outcome research. J Stud Alcohol 2000;61(6):787–93.

20. Dwight-Johnson M, Sherbourne CD, Liao D, et al. Treatment preferences among depressed primary care patients. J Gen Intern Med 2000;15(8):527–34.

21. Andersson G, Cuijpers P. Internet-Based and Other Computerized Psychological Treatments for Adult Depression: A Meta-Analysis. Cogn Behav Ther 2009;38(4): 196–205.

22. Richards D, Richardson T. Computer-based psychological treatments for depression: A systematic review and meta-analysis. Clin Psychol Rev 2012;32(4): 329–42.

23. Cuijpers P, Donker T, van Straten A, et al. Is guided self-help as effective as face-to-face psychotherapy for depression and anxiety disorders? A systematic review

and meta-analysis of comparative outcome studies. Psychol Med 2010;40(12):
1943–57.

24. Linde K, Sigterman K, Kriston L, et al. Effectiveness of Psychological Treatments
for Depressive Disorders in Primary Care: Systematic Review and Meta-Analysis.
Ann Fam Med 2015;13(1):56–68.

25. Wright JH, Mishkind M. Computer-Assisted CBT and Mobile Apps for Depression:
Assessment and Integration Into Clinical Care. FOCUS 2020;18(2):162–8.

26. Donker T, Petrie K, Proudfoot J, et al. Smartphones for Smarter Delivery of Mental
Health Programs: A Systematic Review. J Med Internet Res 2013;15(11):e247.

27. Proudfoot J, Parker G, Hadzi Pavlovic D, et al. Community Attitudes to the Appro-
priation of Mobile Phones for Monitoring and Managing Depression, Anxiety, and
Stress. J Med Internet Res 2010;12(5):e64.

28. Firth J, Torous J, Nicholas J, et al. The efficacy of smartphone-based mental
health interventions for depressive symptoms: a meta-analysis of randomized
controlled trials. World Psychiatry 2017;16(3):287–98.

29. Martínez-Pérez B, de la Torre-Díez I, López-Coronado M. Mobile Health Applications for the Most Prevalent Conditions by the World Health Organization: Review
and Analysis. J Med Internet Res 2013;15(6):e120.

30. Huguet A, Rao S, McGrath PJ, et al. A Systematic review of cognitive behavioral
therapy and behavioral activation apps for depression. In: Choo KKR, editor.
PLoS One 2016;11(5):e0154248. https://doi.org/10.1371/journal.pone.0154248.

31. Seekles W, van Straten A, Beekman A, et al. Stepped care treatment for depression and anxiety in primary care. a randomized controlled trial. Trials 2011;12(1).
https://doi.org/10.1186/1745-6215-12-171.

32. van Straten A, Hill J, Richards DA, et al. Stepped care treatment delivery for
depression: a systematic review and meta-analysis. Psychol Med 2014;45(02):
231–46.

33. Bosmans JE, Dozeman E, van Marwijk HWJ, et al. Cost-effectiveness of a stepped care programme to prevent depression and anxiety in residents in homes
for the older people: a randomised controlled trial. Int J Geriatr Psychiatry
2013;29(2):182–90.

34. van't Veer-Tazelaar P, Smit F, van Hout H, et al. Cost-effectiveness of a stepped
care intervention to prevent depression and anxiety in late life: randomised trial.
Br J Psychiatry 2010;196(4):319–25.

Attention-Deficit/ Hyperactivity Disorder Across the Spectrum
From Childhood to Adulthood

Daniel J. Majarwitz, MD[a], Parvathi Perumareddi, DO[b],*

KEYWORDS

- ADHD • Impulsivity • Hyperactivity • Inattention • Stimulants • Dysregulation
- Neurodevelopmental disorder • Methylphenidate

KEY POINTS

- Attention-deficit hyperactivity disorder is a neurodevelopmental disorder involving dysregulation that manifests in symptoms such as inattention, impulsivity, and hyperactivity. It is most often apparent in childhood revealed through behavior and actions consistent with developmental delays and observed across multiple settings. It persists into adulthood, although symptomology shifts later in life.
- There are often psychiatric comorbidities that should be addressed.
- Diagnosis is a clinical one attained using criteria as set forth in the *Diagnostic and Statistical Manual of Mental Disorders Fifth Edition*.
- Management involves pharmacologic agents such as stimulant or nonstimulant medications, both of which have potential side effects and should be monitored for such. Other nonpharmacologic interventions involve parent and teacher communication, both with each other and the child.

INTRODUCTION

Attention-deficit/hyperactivity disorder (ADHD) is a disorder characterized by an enduring pattern of symptoms that include inattention and/or hyperactivity, leading to disruption of daily functioning. It is one of the most commonly diagnosed neurodevelopmental disorders in the pediatric population, with estimates of 7% to 8% and up to 18% of children in the United States.[1,2] For adults, the estimated prevalence is lower at about 4% to 4.5%, also with a higher incidence among men.[1,3] ADHD manifests in various ways, such as the child having academic problems in school as well as behavioral problems in different

The authors have nothing to disclose.
[a] Department of Psychiatry and Behavioral Medicine, East Carolina University, 905 Johns Hopkins Dr, Greenville, NC 27834, USA; [b] Department of Medicine, Schmidt College of Medicine at Florida Atlantic University, 777 Glades Road, Boca Raton, FL 33431, USA
* Corresponding author.
E-mail address: pperumar@health.fau.edu

Prim Care Clin Office Pract 50 (2023) 21–36
https://doi.org/10.1016/j.pop.2022.10.004
0095-4543/23/© 2023 Elsevier Inc. All rights reserved.

environments and relationship difficulties. Because it persists into adulthood, earlier diagnosis and management is critical for lifelong healthier functioning.

CAUSES

In most cases, it is not known what causes ADHD.[4,5] It is thought that there is a substantial hereditary association secondary to a combination of genetic variants, each contributing to a summative effect.[6,7]

In addition, there is also evidence that environmental factors may be associated with ADHD.[8]

Based on a review of the literature, these risk factors may include the following:

- Peripartum infection (measles, rubella, varicella zoster, encephalitis)[9]
- Extreme birth prematurity or birth weight[10,11]
- Abuse and neglect[10,11]

Almost 30% of children who experience a traumatic brain injury may go on to have ADHD.[12]

PATHOPHYSIOLOGY

ADHD results from neurodevelopmental dysregulation of various circuits. Defects in informational processing in the prefrontal cortex result in executive dysfunction.[13] Specific affected areas include the following:

- Dorsolateral prefrontal cortex ➡ deficits in sustained attention
- Dorsal anterior cingulate cortex ➡ alterations in selective attention and difficulty focusing on tasks
- Orbitofrontal cortex ➡ impulsive symptoms
- Supplementary motor area ➡ motor/hyperactive symptoms.

Other affected regions include the caudate, cerebellum, and parietal lobe.[1,14] Although multiple circuits may be responsible for the symptoms, the commonality seems to be dysregulation of dopamine and norepinephrine neurotransmitters.[1,14] The balance of dopamine and norepinephrine is crucial to proper functioning (**Fig. 1**), and hypoactivity of these catecholamines has traditionally been thought to lead to ADHD symptoms. However, there is some evidence that hyperactivity of these neurons may also play a role.[1] Overall, the imbalance of dopamine and norepinephrine levels in various prefrontal cortex circuits seems to be the main cause of ADHD.

DIAGNOSIS

The defining features of ADHD involve inattention, hyperactivity, and impulsivity. The formal diagnostic criteria can be found in the neurodevelopmental disorder article of the *Diagnostic and Statistical Manual of Mental Disorders Fifth Edition* (DSM-V). **Table 1** shows abbreviated criteria. A patient with ADHD may present with the classical combination of inattention and hyperactivity, but certainly predominately inattentive or predominately hyperactive/impulsive presentations can occur.[15] By definition, symptoms of ADHD must be present before the age of 12 years.[15] That is not to say that ADHD remits or disappears as children grow into adulthood. In fact, symptoms of ADHD often progress, and specific deficits may be more apparent during certain parts of one's life. Hyperactivity and impulsivity are more noticeable during childhood and not as evident in adulthood. Inattention may not be identified during early childhood but becomes more apparent as patients get older, with symptoms persisting into

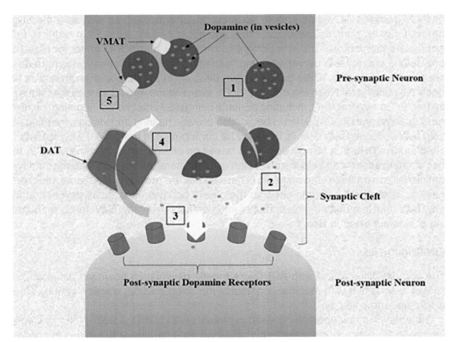

Fig. 1. Depicted is a representation of a neural synapse. (1) Dopamine stored in presynaptic vesicles. (2) Exocytosis of dopamine. (3) Dopamine acts on postsynaptic receptors, leading to downstream cognitive effects. (4) Reuptake of dopamine via the dopamine transporter (DAT) helps to end the transmission. (5) Dopamine transported via vesicular monoamine transporter (VMAT) into vesicles. A similar mechanism exists for norepinephrine and its receptors. In ADHD, catecholamine dysregulation leads to disorganized behavior.

adulthood.[13] It is estimated that 60% to 80% of ADHD symptoms continue into adulthood.[1] Symptoms should be recognized and treated at all stages.

Most cases of ADHD are initially recognized and treated by pediatricians and primary care providers. A thorough history and physical examination is vital in the evaluation of the patient's symptoms. Gathering information regarding the patient's behaviors across

Table 1 Abbreviated attention-deficit/hyperactivity disorder criteria, adapted from the DSM-V	
Inattention	**Hyperactivity**
Careless mistakes	Fidgets
Difficulty sustaining attention	Often leaves seat
Does not seem to listen	Runs/climbs inappropriately
Fails to finish tasks	Cannot quietly engage in activities
Difficulty organizing tasks	"On the go"/"Driven by motor"
Avoids tasks involving sustained effort	Talks excessively
Loses necessary things	Blurts out answers
Easily distracted	Difficulty waiting turn
Forgetful	Interrupts others

Need 6 or more of symptoms in each category for at least 6 months. Must have symptoms before the age of 12 years. Must be in at least 2 settings (ie, school, work, home). Interferes with functioning. Symptoms are not better explained by another psychiatric disorder.

Adapted from American Psychiatric Association. *Diagnostic and Statistical Manual of Mental Disorders.* 5th ed. American Psychiatric Association; 2013.

multiple domains (ie, school, home, extracurricular activities), as well as a thorough medical, family, perinatal/developmental, and social history is crucial in order to fully appreciate risk factors.[16] It is important to remember that ADHD is not localized to one setting but rather is pervasive. A kid "acting up" in school but not elsewhere does not classify as having ADHD but may have difficulty in the particular environment (ie, does the child have a learning disorder?). On examination, providers may see signs of inattention or hyperactivity, including patients being easily distracted, fidgeting, or interrupting conversation. Physicians should also provide hearing and vision screenings to help assess for sensory deficits that may be contributing to the patient's symptoms.[16]

Although ADHD is a clinical diagnosis based on criteria set forth in the DSM-V, the use of rating scales can help the physician gain collateral information that may uncover deficiencies in multiple environments. These scales are provided to patients, teachers, parents, and others who can observe the child's behavior, and these psychometrics may be useful in monitoring response of interventions over time. Several common rating scales are listed in **Box 1**.[1]

COMORBIDITIES

The comorbidities found with ADHD are mostly psychiatric; however, research has shown association with medical conditions, including asthma, obesity, various sleep disorders, and epilepsy.[17,18]

Other psychiatric conditions coexist in patients with ADHD. A 2007 National Center for Health Statistics study collected information from parents or guardians of children in order to assess prevalence of co-occurring disorder. **Fig. 2** lists results from the study.[19] It should be noted that this was a cross-sectional telephone-based survey, in which parents reported whether a doctor or health care provider said that their child had ADHD and other comorbid conditions. A narrative review by Gnanavel and colleagues[20] summarized the rates of the most common comorbid conditions. (**Fig. 3**) Recognition of the extent of comorbid conditions with ADHD is important in order to promptly identify, treat, and refer to a specialist when appropriate.

MANAGEMENT
Pharmacologic Treatment

Before medication initiation, the following should be considered in the baseline assessment[21]:

- Ensuring ADHD criteria for diagnosis are met
- Detailed history, including comorbid psychiatric conditions, substance history, and medical history including medications

---

Box 1
Common rating scales for attention-deficit/hyperactivity disorder

ADHD Symptom Rating Scale

ADHD Rating Scale-IV

Conners Rating Scales—Revised

Inattention/Overactivity with Aggression (IOWA) Conners Teacher Rating Scale

Swanson, Kotkin, Agler, M-Flynn, and Pelham (SKAMP) Rating Scale

Swanson, Nolan, and Pelham-IV (SNAP-IV) Questionnaire

Vanderbilt ADHD Rating Scale

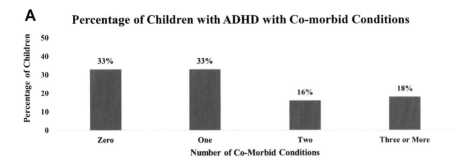

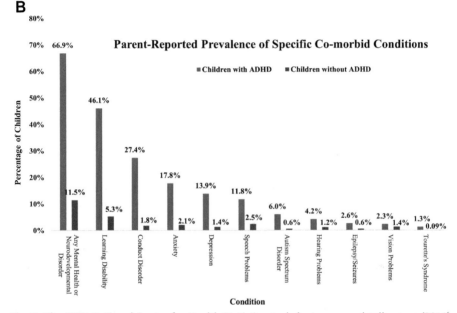

Fig. 2. The 2007 National Center for Health Statistics study by Larson and colleagues (2011) collected data from parent/guardian interviews. Data shown are from the parental reports of whether their children were diagnosed with the condition and not from formal clinical records. (A) Depicted are parent/guardian-reported amount of comorbid conditions in patients with ADHD. (B) Depicted are parent-/guardian-reported prevalence of comorbid conditions in patients with and without ADHD.

- Vitals, including pulse, blood pressure, and height and weight
- Cardiovascular evaluation (electrocardiogram can be considered if patient has increased cardiac risk)
- Cardiology referral for concern related to history of congenital disease, sudden cardiac death of first-degree relative younger than 40 years, palpitations, chest pain, dyspnea on exertion, hypertension, heart failure, or murmur

The origins of ADHD treatment can be traced to the development of the stimulants in the early to mid-twentieth century.[22,23] Although stimulants are the main treatment options for ADHD, nonstimulant medications have also shown efficacy over the years. Newer stimulant medications being developed tend to be manipulations of preexisting mechanisms (ie, delayed release) rather than the formation of drugs of a new class. The main pharmacologic treatment modalities of ADHD are discussed in the following section.

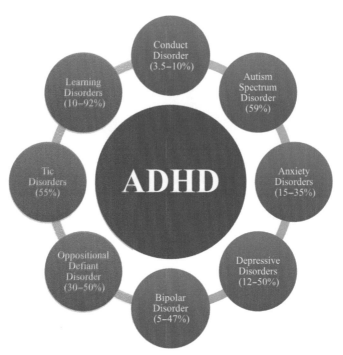

Fig. 3. Listed are the most common comorbid conditions in ADHD with estimated comorbidity rates in parentheses. (*Data from* Gnanavel S, Sharma P, Kaushal P, Hussain S. Attention deficit hyperactivity disorder and comorbidity: A review of literature. World J Clin Cases. 2019;7(17):2420-2426.)

Stimulants

The most used and studied medications for ADHD are stimulants. In general, the stimulant class can be subdivided into the methylphenidate-derived and amphetamine-derived drugs. The goal of these medications is to increase the available dopamine and norepinephrine in the affected neural circuits (**Fig. 4**). For both, the D-isomer is more potent than the L-isomer.[13] Stimulants are listed as Schedule II substances under the Controlled Substances Act due to concerns of abuse.[24]

Common side effects of stimulants include the following:

- Insomnia
- Decreased appetite
- Dry mouth
- Headaches
- Stomach aches
- Tachycardia/Palpitations
- Sweating
- Irritability or dysphoria

Rare side effects include worsening of tics, especially in patients with Tourette syndrome and other tic disorders, as well as changes in mood. If symptoms of psychosis, mania, or depression occur, consider weaning off the medication and referring to a psychiatrist for further evaluation.[25]

Contraindications to stimulant use include the following:

- Active psychosis or mania

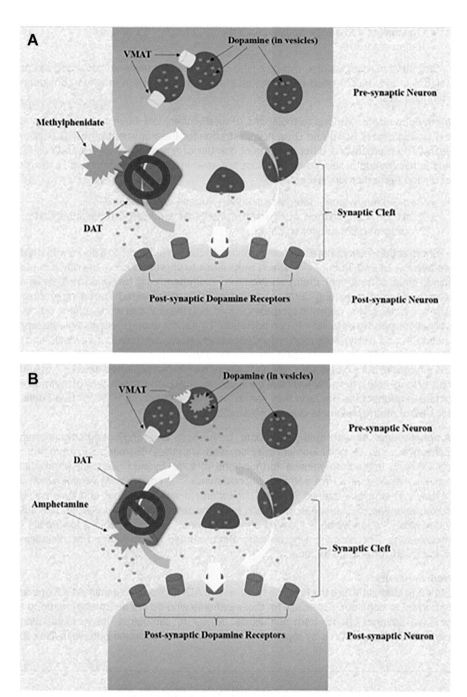

Fig. 4. (A) Methylphenidate and its derivatives increase dopamine and norepinephrine at the synapse by allosterically blocking dopamine transporters (DATs) and norepinephrine transporters (NETs; not shown) on the presynaptic neurons. (B) Amphetamine and its derivatives also block the DATs and NETs (not shown), but unlike methylphenidate, they competitively inhibit the reuptake inhibitors by attaching to the same site that dopamine and

- Concurrent substance abuse
- Eating disorders

Structural cardiac lesions, symptomatic cardiovascular disease, advanced arterio-sclerosis, and uncontrolled hypertension should also be weighed when considering stimulant use.[26,27]

Methylphenidate. Various formulations of methylphenidate have been approved by the United States Food and Drug Administration for the treatment of ADHD over the years. The medications differ in terms of number of active enantiomers and half-life. All methylphenidate-derived medications are used in the racemic form, with a mixture of *d*- and *l*-enantiomers except for[27]

- Two dexmethylphenidate formulations—Focalin and Focalin XR
- Azstarys—combination of dexmethylphenidate and serdexmethylphenidate, a prodrug of dexmethylphenidate[28]

Short-acting methylphenidate has duration of action of around 1 to 5 hours with a half-life average of 2 to 3 hours,[27,29] which limits it use to short periods of the day. For sustained effect of treatment, methylphenidate is recommended to be dosed multiple times a day, or alternatively a long-duration version could be implemented. The timing of administration varies on the patient's symptomology during the day, and work, school, or social obligations need to be taken into consideration. If the short-acting methylphenidate preparation is used, it is typically recommended to start twice a day dose, before meals, and to titrate to effect. Thrice a day dosing can be considered if the medication's effect wanes in the afternoon, but side effects, especially sleep, should be monitored closely.[27,30] A variety of long-acting formulations have been developed to allow for efficacy of methylphenidate throughout the day, and they vary in delivery mechanisms.[25,27,31,36] See **Table 2** for a list of methylphenidate-derived medications.

Amphetamine. As with methylphenidate, both short- and long-acting amphetamine derivatives exist. D- and l-isomers are also used, with the D-isomer being more potent on DATs.[13] Immediate release formulations include Evekeo, Zenzedi (d-amphetamine), Adderall, and ProCentra (d-amphetamine).[13,31] Long-acting versions include Mydayis, Dyanavel, Adzenys, Adderall, Dexedrine (d-amphetamine), and Vyvanse (lisdexamfetamine).[13,31] Lisdexamfetamine is d-amphetamine linked to lysine. It is activated slowly when lysine is cleaved off in the stomach.[13] See **Table 2** for the list of medications. The same dosing considerations should be considered as discussed in the methylphenidate section.

Nonstimulants

Although stimulants are the first-line treatment of ADHD, nonstimulant medications are important to consider, especially for those patients who do not adequately respond to or have adverse effects from stimulants. Similar to stimulants, these medications benefit ADHD symptoms by regulating the central catecholamine pathways (**Box 2**).

---

norepinephrine bind. Amphetamines additionally competitively inhibit the vesicular monoamine transporter (VMAT) and may displace these neurotransmitters from the vesicles (Stahl, 2021). Therefore, by using amphetamine at higher than appropriate doses, the stimulant can be transported into the presynaptic axon and can displace intra-vesicular dopamine into the cytoplasm and then the synapse. This dopamine increase may play a role in the abuse potential and reward pathway of amphetamine (Stahl, 2021).

Table 2
Listed are the Food and Drug Administration–approved medications for the treatment of attention-deficit/hyperactivity disorder

Methylphenidate	Amphetamine
Short-acting	Short-acting
Focalin (tablet)	Adderall (tablet)
Methylphenidate (chewable)	Evekeo (tablet)
Methylin (solution)	Evekeo ODT (orally disintegrating tablet)
Ritalin (tablet)	proCentra (solution)
Long-acting	Zenzedi (tablet)
Adhansia XR (capsule)	Long-acting
Azstarys (capsule)	Adderall XR (capsule)
Aptensio XR (capsule)	Adzenys ER (solution)
Concerta (tablet)	Adzenys XR-ODT (orally disintegrating
Cotempla XR-ODT (orally disintegrating	tablet)
tablet)	Dexedrine Spansule (capsules/tablet)
Daytrana (patch)	Dyanavel (solution)
Focalin XR (capsule)	Mydayis (capsule)
Jornay PM (capsule; dosed in evening)	Vyvanse (capsule)
Metadate CD (capsule)	Vyvanse (chewable)
Metadate ER (tablet)	Nonstimulants
Quillivant ER (chewable)	Guanfacine/Intuniv (tablet)
Quillivant XR (solution)	Clonidine/Kapvay (tablet)
Ritalin (capsule)	Atomoxetine/Straterra (capsule)
	Viloxazine/Qelbree (capsule)

Formulations are listed in parentheses. For a complete, regularly updated list of Food and Drug Administration–approved medications, including the doses and formulations, we recommend the ADHD Medication Guide by Northwell Health.

Data from Adesman A. ADHD Medication Guide. Published October 2021. Accessed April 12, 2022. https://static1.squarespace.com/static/53c961e0e4b06d1cfa9ba29d/t/6172d316f2819837f1979bcc/1634915097746/adhd_med_guide_1021.pdf.

Approach to Pharmacologic Treatment

As discussed earlier, there are a plethora of treatment options available for ADHD, with stimulants being the first-line approach. Treatment of ADHD should be individualized, as patients may respond differently to a particular regimen (ie, stimulant derivative, dose, timing). **Box 3** lists treatment considerations.

The goal of treatment is to find the "sweet spot" in which patients can function and complete tasks during the day while minimizing adverse effects. Long-acting formulations may be preferred by some providers and patients, as these medications can alleviate symptoms throughout the day and minimize interruptions (ie, medication administration during the school day). However, starting with a short-acting stimulant can be considered in order to see efficacy and tolerability; if it does not have benefit or has an adverse effect, the duration will last only a few hours and can be stopped.

In 2018, the National Institute for Health and Care Excellence (NICE) published guidelines regarding the diagnosis and management of ADHD (**Fig. 5**). In a seminal systemic review and meta-analysis study by Cortese and colleagues,[37,38] the investigators looked at 133 double-blind, randomized controlled trials to study the efficacy, tolerability, and acceptability of oral ADHD medications in children, adolescents, and adults (18 years and older). Taking all the information into consideration, the investigators recommended that methylphenidate should be used first line in children and adolescents, whereas amphetamines should be used first line in adults for the short-term

---

Box 2
Nonstimulant medications used to treat attention-deficit/hyperactivity disorder

Atomoxetine (Strattera)
- A selective presynaptic norepinephrine reuptake inhibitor that increases norepinephrine and dopamine in the prefrontal cortex (Banaschewski and colleagues[32], 2004; Stahl [31] 2021).
- FDA-approved inhibitor for children, adolescents, and adults and may help treat comorbid anxiety or depression.
- May be comparable in efficacy with short-acting methylphenidate but not as efficacious as osmotic-release oral methylphenidate (Hanwella and colleagues[33], 2011; Newcorn and colleagues[34], 2008).
- Similar to stimulants, may cause decrease in appetite and weight during initiation.
- No significant cardiovascular effects, including changes in the QTc interval (Banaschewski and colleagues, 2004).

Clonidine (Kapvay)

Guanfacine (Intuniv)
- Alpha-2 adrenergic agonists
- FDA-approved medications and modulate norepinephrine in various brain regions including prefrontal cortex, posterior parietal cortex, and locus ceruleus (Banaschewski and colleagues, 2004; Stahl [31] 2021).
- Can be used as adjunct with stimulants, especially to help with sleep, tics, or aggressive behavior.
- This class, but especially clonidine, can affect blood pressure and heart conduction, as well as cause somnolence.
- Guanfacine causes less sedation than clonidine and should be considered for daytime use if needed.

Viloxazine (Qelbree)
- Novel ADHD agent
- FDA-approved in 2021 for ADHD for children 6 to 17 years old (Food and Drug Administration, 04/21; Lamb[35], 2021).
- Inhibits the norepinephrine reuptake transporters.
- Side effects include somnolence, decreased appetite, headache, and insomnia (Food and Drug Administration, 04/21; Lamb, 2021).

Bupropion (Wellbutrin)
- A norepinephrine and dopamine reuptake inhibitor that can be used off-label for ADHD (Banaschewski and colleagues, 2004).
- Shown to improve ADHD symptoms but overall seems less effective than stimulants.
- Also used to treat comorbid depression.
- Side effects include insomnia, headache, nausea, dry mouth, drowsiness, and may make tics worse.
- Should be avoided for those with coexisting seizure disorder, as well as current or previous eating disorder (Food and Drug Administration,[36] 2017b).
- Contraindicated in the setting of abrupt cessation of alcohol, benzodiazepines/barbiturates, or antiepileptic medication (Food and Drug Administration,[36] 2017b).

Tricyclic Antidepressants (TCAs)
- Affect norepinephrine and dopamine reuptake.
- Used off-label to treat ADHD (Banaschewski and colleagues, 2004).
- Evidence has shown benefit, in particular desipramine, compared with placebo, but as a class TCAs may not be effective as stimulants (Banaschewski and colleagues, 2004).
- Because of the side effects (including cardiovascular effects) and narrow safety profile, TCAs are not routinely considered for treatment of ADHD.

---

treatment of ADHD.[37] However, this study was multifaceted, and it is recommended to refer to the article for specific drug comparisons and adverse effects. Overall, there are quite a few factors to consider as mentioned; therefore, treatment for ADHD should be tailored to the individual patient (**Fig. 6**).

> **Box 3**
> **Attention-deficit/hyperactivity disorder treatment should be individualized, with the aforementioned factors taken into consideration**
>
> Treatment considerations when using stimulants
>   Stimulant class
>   Formulation (ie, short- vs long-acting)
>   Dose
>   Timing
>   Augmenting agents (use of nonstimulants)
>
> Consider switching stimulant classes if the patient does not seem to be benefiting from a particular derivative (ie, methylphenidate versus amphetamine). Providers should monitor for reoccurrence of symptoms during the day and if present, should consider dose adjustments or adding a short-acting stimulant to continue effect. It is important to assess whether the adverse effects happen acutely (within a few hours of administration) or when the medication is wearing off, as the timing of symptoms will guide whether to reduce the dose or change the formulation (ie, short- to long-acting). If insomnia ensues, consider moving the dose earlier in the afternoon (ie, before 6 pm) and/or lowering the dose. If ADHD symptoms seem present later in the day, suggesting a wear-off period, then it may be necessary to switch to a long-acting version or add a short-acting stimulant to maintain effect. Providers should also monitor for worsening symptoms, including cognitive dysfunction, if the stimulant dose is increased too much.

Recommendations for Monitoring

For patients taking medications for ADHD, it is important to regularly monitor vitals.

- Consider measuring height for children and young people every 6 months.
- For children 10 years and younger, consider measuring weight every 3 months.
- For patients older than 10 years and adolescents, consider measuring weight at 3 and 6 months after treatment and then every 6 months or more often if needed.
- Plotting height and weight on a growth chart is important to monitor for any deviations.
- For adults, consider obtaining weights every 6 months.
- Obtain pulse and blood pressure every 6 months and before and after any dose adjustments.

If patient has tachycardia, arrythmia, or blood pressure greater than 95th percentile or clinically significant increase measured on 2 occasions, then consider reducing the dose and referring for evaluation. If tics occur, assess whether they are in relationship to the medication and assess the risks versus benefits of ADHD treatment. If tics are related to the stimulant, consider reducing dose or changing to a nonstimulant, such as atomoxetine, guanfacine, or clonidine. Monitor for any sleep disturbances and adjust dose or timing of medication. Monitor for any sexual dysfunction (ie, with atomoxetine), new or worsening seizures, and worsening behavior when ADHD medication is started, and adjust medications as appropriate.[21]

Nonpharmacologic Treatment

Psychosocial interventions may play a helpful role in the management of ADHD. Because this disorder involves behavioral disturbances, it is important that both the child's parents/caregivers and school teachers/officials be educated and familiar with the condition, including knowledge of the child's abilities, what is in their control, and how best to manage the behavior patterns. Two important aspects to focus on involve communication and problem-solving skills.

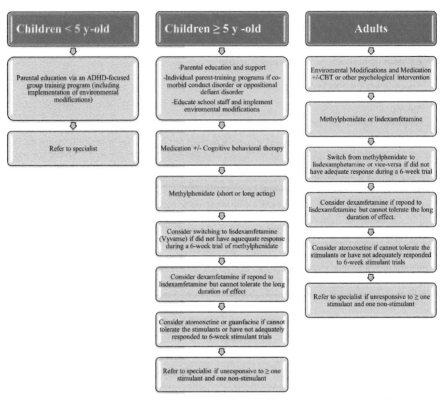

Fig. 5. Treatment algorithm according to the 2018 National Institute for Health and Care Excellence (NICE) guidelines. Environment modifications depend on the individual circumstances and should be tailored to the patient. Examples include adjusting lighting and noise, using headphones to reduce distractions, changing seating arrangements, encouraging frequent breaks, and having shorter episodes where focus is needed, and having breaks. Please refer to the NICE Web site for more details regarding management options. This algorithm is one of many; as previously discussed, there are many approaches to treating ADHD, and a customized plan should be implemented for each patient.

The groundbreaking Multimodal Treatment Study of Children with ADHD (MTA) study in the 1990s looked at 579 children between 7 and 10 years old.[34] The study showed that medication management was superior to behavioral intervention and that combined treatment of medication and behavioral therapy did not show significantly greater benefit than medication alone in terms of alleviating core ADHD symptoms.[34] Other studies have shown that behavioral interventions may be as

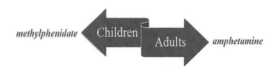

Fig. 6. Cortese and colleagues (2019) reviewed 133 double-blinded, randomized controlled trials in order to assess various ADHD medications. Considering efficacy and safety profiles, the investigators recommended using methylphenidate in children/adolescents and amphetamines in adults as preferred first-line medications for short-term management of ADHD.

efficacious as low-dose stimulants and thus can be considered if mild symptoms are present.[1]

Important behavioral interventions to implement include the following[16]:

- Parent training/education, which may use rewards to target good behaviors and tactics to minimize disruptive behaviors.
  - Sessions can be done individually or in groups.
- Peer interventions involve training skills to help with social interactions.
- Classroom management involves providing a structured environment and routine to help minimize negative behaviors and highlight positive ones.
  - For example, the use of a token economy operantly reinforces the positive behaviors, and daily report cards can share feedback to the child and parents.

Modifications to address the patient's response to stimuli may include the following[39]:

- Breaking down tasks into smaller ones
- Setting short periods of time to work on tasks to enhance focus
- Repeating instructions often for a given task
- Altering presentation of task instructions to make it more interesting
- Using enthusiasm or rewards/tokens to encourage the child

There is thought that exercise may aid short term in the management of ADHD in conjunction with stimulant medications due to effects of norepinephrine and dopamine.[40] Parents and teachers have reported reduced symptoms and improved social and classroom behavior.[40]

Overall, behavioral interventions are an important component to the management of ADHD, but medications should also be used. Although these behavioral techniques are not proved superior to pharmacologic treatments, they may useful adjunctively. A multimodal approach is often necessary and maintained over time.[39] Healthychildren.org provides some tips that may help parents with addressing behavioral issues[41] (**Table 3**).

Table 3
Techniques to help address behavioral disturbances

Technique	Description	Intervention
Positive reinforcement	Complimenting and providing rewards to achieve desired behavior	Child completes task and is allowed to participate in play activity they like
Time out	Removing child from activity because of undesirable behavior	Child screams and as a result must sit in a time out for several minutes
Response cost	Privileges or rewards are withdrawn because of unwanted behavior	Child loses activity they like because of not completing assigned tasks
Token economy	Combining reward and consequences. Child earns behavior and privileges when they participate in desired behavior. They lose rewards and privileges when they participate in undesired behavior	Child earns points, token, or stars for completing tasks (ie, schoolwork) and loses points for getting out of seat. Child can accumulate and trade points for a prize at the end of a specified time period

Data from Barkley RA. Psychosocial treatments for attention-deficit/hyperactivity disorder in children. J Clin Psychiatry. 2002;63 Suppl 12:36-43.

FUTURE DIRECTION

Some research has been conducted on measurement of biomarkers, which may be helpful in diagnosis of ADHD. These biomarkers include urinary phenethylamine, urinary 3-methoxy-4-hydroxyphenylethylene glycol, urinary norepinephrine, and platelet monoamine oxidase. However, further studies are necessary to determine definitive correlation as well as clinical significance.[42]

CLINICS CARE POINTS

- Consider ADHD in the differential diagnosis for children who shows signs of disinhibition, inattention, or hyperactivity.
- Symptoms are beyond the control of the child and should not be perceived as "bad" behavior.
- Impulsivity and hyperactivity tend to decline by early adulthood, whereas inattention persists. Furthermore, comorbid conditions may become more apparent as patients age.
- Testing for diagnosis can be done by a primary care physician, pediatrician, psychologist, or psychiatrist and is achieved through DSM criteria.
- Parents, teachers, school officials, and the primary care providers all play a role in treatment of the child. In addition, there are circumstances in which a psychologist or psychiatrist may be a part of the interdisciplinary team both for prescribing medications as well as providing counseling for both the child and the parents.
- There are various rating scales that can be used to obtain information regarding behavior and response to interventions across multiple settings.
- Stimulants are considered first-line therapy, but nonstimulants may be used as adjuncts or if patients cannot tolerate side effects of stimulants.
- Monitoring vitals and adverse effects of pharmacologic agents is necessary.
- Nonpharmacologic interventions involve caregiver education, behavioral modifications for the child, and close communication between parents and teachers.
- The treatment plan should be individualized for the patient, as no one size fits all.
- Because ADHD is lifelong and can affect various parts of cognition and behavior, early treatment is crucial to help improve overall functioning.

REFERENCES

1. Sharma A, Couture J. A Review of the Pathophysiology, Etiology, and Treatment of Attention-Deficit Hyperactivity Disorder (ADHD). Ann Pharmacother 2014;48(2): 209–25.
2. Wetterer L. Attention-Deficit/Hyperactivity Disorder: AAP Updates Guideline for Diagnosis and Management. Am Fam Physician 2020;102(1):58–60.
3. Kessler RC, Adler L, Barkley R, et al. The prevalence and correlates of adult ADHD in the United States: results from the National Comorbidity Survey Replication. Am J Psychiatry 2006;163(4):716–23.
4. Franke B, Michelini G, Asherson P, et al. Live fast, die young? A review on the developmental trajectories of ADHD across the lifespan. Eur Neuropsychopharmacol 2018;28(10):1059–88.
5. Attention-Deficit/Hyperactivity Disorder in Children and Teens: What You Need to Know. National Institute of Mental Health (NIMH). Available at: https://www.nimh.

nih.gov/health/publications/attention-deficit-hyperactivity-disorder-in-children-and-teens-what-you-need-to-know. Accessed May 12, 2022.

6. Faraone SV, Larsson H. Genetics of attention deficit hyperactivity disorder. Mol Psychiatry 2019;24(4):562–75.

7. Faraone SV, Banaschewski T, Coghill D, et al. The World Federation of ADHD International Consensus Statement: 208 Evidence-based Conclusions about the Disorder. Neurosci Biobehav Rev 2021;128:789–818.

8. CDC. Research on ADHD | CDC. Centers for Disease Control and Prevention. 2020. Available at: https://www.cdc.gov/ncbddd/adhd/research.html. Accessed May 12, 2022.

9. Millichap JG. Etiologic Classification of Attention-Deficit/Hyperactivity Disorder. Pediatrics 2008;121(2):e358–65.

10. Thapar A, Cooper M, Jefferies R, et al. What causes attention deficit hyperactivity disorder? Arch Dis Child 2012;97(3):260–5.

11. Botting N, Powls A, Cooke RWI, et al. Attention Deficit Hyperactivity Disorders and Other Psychiatric Outcomes in Very Low Birthweight Children at 12 Years. J Child Psychol Psychiatry 1997;38(8):931–41.

12. Eme R. ADHD: an integration with pediatric traumatic brain injury. Expert Rev Neurother 2012;12(4):475–83.

13. Stahl SM. Stahl's essential psychopharmacology: neuroscientific basis and practical applications. 5th ed. Cambridge University Press; 2021. https://doi.org/10.1017/9781108975292.

14. Vance A, Silk TJ, Casey M, et al. Right parietal dysfunction in children with attention deficit hyperactivity disorder, combined type: a functional MRI study. Mol Psychiatry 2007;12(9):826–32.

15. American Psychiatric Association. Diagnostic and statistical manual of mental disorders. 5th edition. Washington, DC: American Psychiatric Association; 2013.

16. Felt BT, Biermann B, Christner JG, et al. Diagnosis and Management of ADHD in Children. Am Fam Physician 2014;90(7):456–64.

17. Instanes JT, Klungsøyr K, Halmøy A, et al. Adult ADHD and Comorbid Somatic Disease: A Systematic Literature Review. J Atten Disord 2018;22(3):203–28.

18. NHS. Attention deficit hyperactivity disorder (ADHD) - Symptoms. nhs.uk. 2021. Available at: https://www.nhs.uk/conditions/attention-deficit-hyperactivity-disorder-adhd/symptoms/. Accessed May 12, 2022.

19. Larson K, Russ SA, Kahn RS, et al. Patterns of Comorbidity, Functioning, and Service Use for US Children With ADHD, 2007. Pediatrics 2011;127(3):462–70.

20. Gnanavel S, Sharma P, Kaushal P, et al. Attention deficit hyperactivity disorder and comorbidity: A review of literature. World J Clin Cases 2019;7(17):2420–6.

21. NICE Guidelines - Attention deficit hyperactivity disorder: diagnosis and management. 2018. Available at: https://www.nice.org.uk/guidance/ng87. Accessed March 1, 2022.

22. Heal DJ, Smith SL, Gosden J, et al. Amphetamine, past and present – a pharmacological and clinical perspective. J Psychopharmacol Oxf Engl 2013;27(6):479–96.

23. Morton WA, Stockton GG. Methylphenidate Abuse and Psychiatric Side Effects. Prim Care Companion J Clin Psychiatry 2000;2(5):159–64.

24. Controlled Substance Schedules. Available at: https://www.deadiversion.usdoj.gov/schedules/. Accessed January 23, 2022.

25. Stevens JR, Wilens TE, Stern TA. Using Stimulants for Attention-Deficit/Hyperactivity Disorder: Clinical Approaches and Challenges. Prim Care Companion CNS Disord 2013;15(2):12f01472. PCC.

26. Food and Drug Administration. Adderall. FDA Label. 2007. Available at: https://www.accessdata.fda.gov/drugsatfda_docs/label/2017/011522s043lbl.pdf. Accessed March 1, 2022.

27. McVoy M, Findling R. Clinical manual of child and adolescent psychopharmacology. Third. Arlington, VA: American Psychiatric Association Publishing; 2017.

28. Food and Drug Administration. Azstarys. HIGHLIGHTS OF PRESCRIBING INFORMATION. 2021. Available at: https://www.accessdata.fda.gov/drugsatfda_docs/label/2021/212994s000lbl.pdf. Accessed March 1, 2022.

29. Kimko HC, Cross JT, Abernethy DR. Pharmacokinetics and Clinical Effectiveness of Methylphenidate. Clin Pharmacokinet 1999;37(6):457–70.

30. Food and Drug Administration. RITALIN and RITALIN-SR. HIGHLIGHTS OF PRESCRIBING INFORMATION. 2019. Available at: https://www.accessdata.fda.gov/drugsatfda_docs/label/2019/010187s071s082,018029s041s051lbl.pdf. Accessed March 1, 2022.

31. Adesman A. ADHD Medication Guide. 2021. Available at: https://static1.squarespace.com/static/53c961e0e4b06d1cfa9ba29d/t/6172d316f2819837f1979bcc/1634915097746/adhd_med_guide_1021.pdf. Accessed April 12, 2022.

32. Banaschewski T, Roessner V, Dittmann RW, et al. Non–stimulant medications in thetreatment of ADHD. European Child & Adolescent Psychiatry 2004;13(1):i102–16. https://doi.org/10.1007/s00787-004-1010-x.

33. Hanwella R, Senanayake M, de Silva V. Comparative efficacy and acceptability of methylphenidate and atomoxetine in treatment of attention deficit hyperactivity disorder in children and adolescents: A meta-analysis. BMC Psychiatry 2011;11(1):176. https://doi.org/10.1186/1471-244X-11-176.

34. Newcorn JH, Kratochvil CJ, Allen AJ, et al. Atomoxetine and Osmotically Released Methylphenidate for the Treatment of Attention Deficit Hyperactivity Disorder: Acute Comparison and Differential Response. American Journal of Psychiatry 2008;165(6):721–30. https://doi.org/10.1176/appi.ajp.2007.05091676.

35. Lamb YN. Viloxazine: Pediatric First Approval. Pediatric Drugs 2021;23(4):403–9. https://doi.org/10.1007/s40272-021-00453-3.

36. Food and Drug Administration. Concerta. HIGHLIGHTS OF PRESCRIBING INFORMATION. 2017. Available at: https://www.accessdata.fda.gov/drugsatfda_docs/label/2017/021121s038lbl.pdf. Accessed March 1, 2022.

37. Cortese S, Adamo N, Giovane CD, et al. Comparative efficacy and tolerability of medications for attention-deficit hyperactivity disorder in children, adolescents, and adults: a systematic review and network meta-analysis. Lancet Psychiatry 2018;5(9):727–38.

38. The MTA Cooperative Group. A 14-Month Randomized Clinical Trial of Treatment Strategies for Attention-Deficit/Hyperactivity Disorder. Arch Gen Psychiatry 1999;56(12):1073–86.

39. Barkley RA. Psychosocial treatments for attention-deficit/hyperactivity disorder in children. J Clin Psychiatry 2002;63(Suppl 12):36–43.

40. Den Heijer AE, Groen Y, Tucha L, et al. Sweat it out? The effects of physical exercise on cognition and behavior in children and adults with ADHD: a systematic literature review. J Neural Transm 2017;124(Suppl 1):3–26.

41. HealthyChildren.org - From the American Academy of Pediatrics. HealthyChildren.org. Available at: https://healthychildren.org/English/Pages/default.aspx. Accessed May 11, 2022.

42. Scassellati C, Bonvicini C, Faraone SV, et al. Biomarkers and Attention-Deficit/Hyperactivity Disorder: A Systematic Review and Meta-Analyses. J Am Acad Child Adolesc Psychiatry 2012;51(10):1003–19.e20.

Perils and Pitfalls of Social Media Use
Cyber Bullying in Teens/Young Adults

Jennifer Caceres, MD, Allison Holley, MD*

KEYWORDS

- Social media • Cyberbullying • Mental health • Technology • Internet user • Bullying
- Adolescent health

KEY POINTS

- Social media has become a social norm and its integration into daily life necessitates recognition of the potential impact on adolescent development. Health care providers and parents must take an active role in monitoring the use of social media of children and adolescents.
- Most of the adolescents and young adults have experienced bullying in some form, with about one-third of these experiencing cyberbullying, contributing to mental health concerns.
- Primary-care physicians should screen adolescents and young adults for inappropriate or misuse of social media and cyberbullying using a screening tool developed for use in the health care setting.
- Counseling interventional programs and educational programs can be used through the school system or community groups to help prevent cyberbullying and treat those who have been affected by it.

HISTORY

Social media has become a social norm and its integration into the daily life stems from networked communication that evolved into platformer sociality. In 1991, the World Wide Web was invented to create networked media, including Weblogs and e-mail services supporting online and offline communities. However, it did not automatically connect people to others. Then came Web 2.0 where the opportunity for exchange of communication and creative content among "friends" began and the development of platforms for sociality was born. Social media started as informal and transient expressions of social interaction, but has gradually transitioned into a forum of socialization with far-reaching and long-lasting effects. Social media

Florida Atlantic University Schmidt College of Medicine, 777 Glades Road BC-71, Boca Raton, FL 33431, USA
* Corresponding author.
E-mail address: holleya@health.fau.edu

Prim Care Clin Office Pract 50 (2023) 37–45
https://doi.org/10.1016/j.pop.2022.10.008
primarycare.theclinics.com

platforms have now changed what was once a conversation between a selected few to public communication among "friends."[1]

It is important for parents and health care providers to understand how social media is now programmed to best understand the potential impacts of social media on children and adolescents. The initial platforms created were designed to transmit communication and information among its users, but over time the focus shifted to emphasize user-generated information and applied services. Social media platforms are no longer a generic conduit to share information, but rather a programmed application with specific objectives. It is the understanding of how these platforms have now infiltrated the daily and hourly lives of our children and how it is programmed that may influence their developing minds. Social media platforms are no longer finished products being offered to users. Instead, it is now a dynamic tool of communication that responds to the users' needs, but also the owner's objectives within competing platforms and larger technological and economic infrastructures. These programmed objectives can leave adolescents susceptible to overuse or addictive behaviors of social media.

INTRODUCTION

Social media use among adolescents has benefits as well as risks. Adolescents and young adults use social media and technology for numerous applications. Positive uses of this technology can include working together on homework or class projects, connecting with peers, scheduling events, using health apps that encourage healthy lifestyles, providing support, interacting with family members that are separated geographically, and connecting teens with disabilities. There are also concerning negative characteristics of technology including the fact that heavy utilization is linked to mental health disorders including depression, anxiety, and attention disorders, as well as decreased life satisfaction, and diminished ability to connect in face-to-face interactions.[2] With the increase use on what may no longer be a mere daily basis, but rather an hourly or even more frequent basis among adolescents, parents and health care providers must play a more active role in monitoring its use and recognize potential positive and negative long-term impacts.

Why do so many adolescents gravitate toward social media? An important aspect of adolescent development is the formation of close and meaningful relationships and social media provides a method for adolescents to form more new relationships while maintaining and strengthening existing ones.[3] Social media also produces an opportunity for those who want to overcome shyness to develop new relationships because of some degree of anonymity that it offers compared with face-to-face interactions. This may allow them to test the waters and gain confidence to further develop a social network.[4] Social media may also help teens connect with those with common interests, allowing them to further develop their specific hobbies. It also provides a platform for teens to express their creativity and share their talents,[3] helping them develop their self-identity. In addition, social media can provide useful educational resources that can be easily accessed by teens and serve as a tool to deliver information on healthy and safe life choices.

It is clear that there are aspects of social media that are beneficial to adolescents, however, as teens explore their identity, including their sexuality, there is the potential for display of risky behavior such as posting images, videos, or texts related to sex, drugs, and violence. They may even post content pictures of themselves participating in risky or illegal behaviors without the awareness or understanding of the potential consequences of such actions.[5] Sexting, sending or receiving of sexually explicit or sexually suggestive images, can easily become disseminated even if initially sent privately to only one person. This type of dissemination of sensitive and explicit images may lead to harassment or cyberbullying, significantly impacting the mental health and well-being of adolescents.[6]

Looking beyond display of risky behaviors and its consequences, the constant availability of social media may also amplify the expectations of accessibility by friends leading to peer pressure to constantly be available.[7] Moreover cyberbullying, defined as "willful and repeated harm inflicted through the use of computers, cell phones, and other electronic devices,"[8] can have even farther-reaching impacts than traditional bullying due to the degree of anonymity social media affords users and the increased amount of time available to expose teens to cyberbullying. This has resulted in concerns of increased rates of mental health issues, including suicide. Furthermore, although social media may increase accessibility to information and education, it also increases access to misinformation and misuse of information, including those found on pro-self-harm and pro-eating disorder websites.

Adolescents are reporting some of these negative consequences, with 34% of teenagers feeling that social media distracts them from spending time with people in person, and 44% feeling that social media diverted their attention away from people they were previously spending time with.[2] These negative effects can be more complex in that some studies have shown the outcomes of technology use are linked to the type of content viewed, the type and amount of information disclosed, the quality of the interactions, and the reactions of their peers to content posted.[2] There has also been debate on whether social media use promotes or diminishes adolescents ability to empathize with others. Some studies feel that social media and technology use have partially contributed to the decline in empathy among young adults.[9] Another study argues that social media use can promote the development of empathy over time. In this study, over 900 Dutch adolescents were surveyed on two separate occasions with a year in between the survey. In the survey, participants recorded the number of days and time they spent on social media, and the AMES (Adolescent Measure of Empathy and Sympathy) was administered, and the results show that both cognitive and affective empathy were improved by social media use.[10]

CLINICAL RELEVANCE
What is the impact of social media use/cyberbullying on mental health issues?

Cyberbullying is defined as bullying by the use of electronic communication which can include texts, emails, online videos, social media, forums, blogs, message boards, and numerous other types of electronic media. It has become much more of a problem over the last few decades, and several reasons for this include the anonymity it allows, the fact that it is not as easily monitored, and adolescents and young adults have easier access to devices.[11] According to the Cyberbullying Research Center's research by Drs. Hinduja and Patchin, 75% of teens ages 12 to 17 have been a victim of bullying with 30% being victims of cyberbullying, and in the 9 to 12 age group, almost 15% had been a victim of cyberbullying.[12] The CDC also shows similar statistics with 14.9% of high-school students experiencing cyberbullying.[13] Most teens and young adults are constantly connected to devices, putting them at a constant risk of victimization at all hours of the day and night.[12] More than 75% of teenagers have cell phones, and on average, they send at least 60 text messages per day,[11] and 43% report using social media on a daily basis with an average of 2 h time spent.[2]

Some of the risk factors for being a victim of cyberbullying include low self-esteem, anxiety, stress, suicidal ideation, reduced levels of empathy or social intelligence, high technology usage, being a part of a single-parent household, negative home life experience, sexual abuse, and having been a victim of traditional bullying. Protective factors include low technology use, ability to effectively regulate emotions, social awareness, family support, parental supervision of technology, and high socioeconomic status.[13]

Social media use may contribute to feelings of anxiety as many teens report that being able to follow or see their peers' daily life often minute by minute can leave them with "FOMO" (feelings of missing out) prompting teens into thinking that their peers are living more fulfilled, interesting, fun lives and that their inability to match this can cause anxiety and trigger further social media use. Teens also have an increased risk of mood disorders due to lack of sleep due to staying on social media late into the night. About 20% of teens wake up at night to check social media messages, which obviously impairs their sleep. Many teens also have multiple social media accounts, which can further increase anxiety by encouraging them to craft a specific online identity on each platform. Some adolescents and young adults develop problematic Internet use (PUI) or Internet and video game addiction (IVGA) which both involve the inability to self-regulate how much time they spend on Internet and the development of anxiety and distress when their devices or Internet are not available. A need for social assurance or affirmation is more likely to predispose an adolescent or young adult to social media addiction as people are affected differently by social media and technology habits and use. This can lead to a cycle of anxiety stemming from predisposition to or already diagnosed anxiety → that leads to further social media use → which can lead to overuse → which can decrease sleep → which in turn worsens mood → impacting overall mental health.[14]

In one study, more than 6,000 students ages 11 to 18 participated in a self-reported survey collected in 2019, and in this questionnaire, it was found that 17% had been victims of cyberbullying and 10% had been perpetrators of cyberbullying. It also discovered that bullying in any form, either as a victim or a perpetrator, was linked to depression, anxiety, and engagement in self-harm with girls being more likely to have poor mental health outcomes.[15] The Youth Risk Behavior Surveillance System which is sponsored by the CDC has found that 18% of US high-school students have suicidal ideation. According to a 2014 meta-analysis of nearly 285,000 adolescents, suicidal ideation is directly linked to peer victimization.[16,17] Teenage girls experience cyberbullying at a rate of 36% versus 30% in teenage boys, members of minority groups experience cyberbullying at much higher rates at 49%[11] and members of the LGBTQ + community report cyberbullying at a rate of 27% compared with 13% in their heterosexual peers.[17] Teenage girls are also more likely to be victims of cyber sexual harassment. A study of teenage girls that were patients of an urban San Diego clinic revealed that 68.6% had experienced some form of cyber sexual harassment, and cyber sexual harassment was linked to increase in depression, anxiety, suicidal thoughts, alcohol use, and drug use.[18] A longitudinal retrospective study was performed that spanned five decades included more than 18,000 participants born in 1958 in England, Scotland, and Wales who were surveyed over the course of five decades at ages 7, 11, 16, 23, 33, 42, 45, and 50 years old. This study found that being a victim of bullying increased the use of mental health services compared with those not bullied and this was true for ages 16 to 50 years old, with the highest utilization at age 16 which is assumed to be the age closest to the bullying victimization event.[19]

What can primary-care physicians do?

As primary-care physicians, it is our job to screen and evaluate for things that can do our patients harm. This duty includes screening for social media use, bullying/

cyberbullying, mental health issues, as well as countless others. Only half of health care providers who see pediatric patients were found to be consistently screening for bullying.[20] Part of this may be because there are not many screening tools for these issues specifically designed for health care settings. A few of the screening tools that can be used include the Revised Olweus Bully/Victim Questionnaire (R-OBVQ), the California Bullying Victimization Scale (CBVS), and the Child Adolescent Bullying Scale (CABS).[21] The Massachusetts Aggression Reduction Center (MARC) and the Bullying and Cyberbullying Prevention and Advocacy Collaborative has a helpful screening tool for bullying and cyberbullying checklist that physicians can use during patient visits. This checklist form can be found at https://www.marccenter.org/resources-for-practitioners.[22] A screening tool of the providers' choice should be worked into the work-flow of pediatric visits to ensure that screening is consistently done and results are addressed in a timely manner. MARC also offers a program with advice on the best way to deal with bullying including cyberbullying that will be discussed further in the section on community and school programs.

To screen for technology and social media use, physicians can easily ask parents or the patient themselves (1) How many hours per day are spent on screens of any kind? and (2) Is there a television or other device with Internet access in the bedroom? To screen for cyberbullying or bullying of any kind, physicians can also ask patients if they feel safe at school, home, and online, and have they ever experienced bullying or cyberbullying either themselves or someone they know.[23]

Physicians can also ask about the many symptoms that could be warnings signs of cyberbullying such as sleep disorders, mood disorders, eating disorders, suicidal thoughts, self-harm behaviors, academic problems, fatigue, and headaches. Physicians can also undergo training to detect bullying and ensure that their staff is trained appropriately. Making sure to establish community contacts with groups and organizations such as local schools, law enforcement, mental health counselors specializing in trauma care, suicide prevention groups, and patient and family support groups that can provide services for prevention, screening, and victim support services also are crucial to helping patients. Posters in the waiting room or exam rooms or helpline numbers can also help to education patients and their families on how to prevent and deal with cyberbullying. A valid resource for these materials with practical tips on addressing this issue in your practice can be found at cyberbullying.org, a cyber-bullying research center.[12]

What can parents and family members do?

A staggering statistic in regards to the reporting of cyberbullying found that only 23% of students who were cyberbullied reported it to an adult at their school which shows that many incidences go unreported which is another crucial reason to screen patients as well as to educate parents. A variety of reasons for this exist, including that teens do not want to report due to the feeling that they should deal with this on their own and due to fear of repercussions including getting their devices are taken away or restrictions on Internet or phone usage.[11] When educating parents about cyberbullying, it is important to establish it as a health concern rather than a social problem. This can help parents better understand the implications it may have rather than chalking it up to normal teenage behavior that will resolve on its own.[12] As one of the best protective factors in cyberbullying is having a social support system,[11] it is important that parents keep open lines of communication with their children as well as validating their feelings to better facilitate screening, preventing, and dealing with any cyberbullying. Parents must also teach their children about appropriate online behavior, set boundaries, and give clear guidelines with appropriate consequences for rule-breaking. Boundaries to set can include not posting personal information, not sharing login information such as usernames and passwords, not responding to inappropriate messages, turning off technology if these type of messages are received, and immediately reporting an incident to an adult.[24] When an incident does occur, rather than engaging the cyberbully in further communication to discuss the incident, which has been found to make it worse, it is recommended to block the cyberbully and report the incident to the appropriate social media source.[13] Teens must also understand that access to technology, devices, and social media is a privilege that is earned through trust and not simply an inherent right.[25]

Parents often find it difficult to know what are the appropriate uses of technology, what are the normal time parameters, and what are the relevant consequences for rule violations. These are often difficult for parents because every family situation should be individualized to their needs. Setting clear, defined, simple expectations is key. A few areas that can be included in setting clear limits and expectations include technology hours allowed per day, allowing for tech-free family time, location of devices, and media usage such as in shared common areas rather than in bedrooms. Active monitoring rather than solely restrictive monitoring is generally the approach recommended by experts in this field. Active monitoring techniques for parents can include viewing media with their teens or actively discussing what types of media, apps, websites, and games they like to use and what they like about them and keeping updated on the new apps that are regularly coming out.

Several organizations have online resources for parents such as Cyberwise (cyberwise.org), Common Sense Media (commonsensemedia.org), and Plugged In (pluggedin.com) among others. The American Academy of Pediatrics offers online digital media contracts for families to individualize and use that can be found at https://www.healthychildren.org/English/family-life/Media/Pages/How-to-Make-a-Family-Media-Use-Plan.aspx (accessed April 29, 2022).[26] Finally, the American Academy of Child & Adolescent Psychiatry has a section on Facts for Families on many different topics http://www.aacap.org/AACAP/Families_and_Youth/Facts_for_Families/FFF-Guide/FFF-Guide-Home.aspx (accessed April 20, 2022).[27] Parents can also model healthy media behavior by following similar rules themselves and developing alternative coping mechanisms and healthy habits to avoid the use of devices in children's bedtimes routines, to please a crying child, or as a babysitter to young children for them to be able to accomplish household chores.[28]

What can the community do?

Counseling interventional programs and educational programs can be used through the school system or community groups to help prevent cyberbullying and treat those who have been affected by it. The focus of these programs should be to teach coping mechanisms, to encourage people to speak up when they are being cyberbullied or see someone else being cyberbullied,[15] and to teach students how to regulate their emotions and control their anger.[29] Some of the traditional ways in which we deal with conflict resolution in the school system may be making cyberbullying worse. Educators and counselors in the school system often use techniques such as mediation and negotiation. This may work well for other types of behaviors and are effective discipline technique for other problems, but cyberbullying may be made worse by using these techniques for several reasons. In mediation, the assumption is that the power dynamic is equal and the involved parties are willing to discuss and recognize the other person's point of view which are not usually the case in a bullying situation. Instead, research has discovered that setting limits and being consistent with the enforcement of these limits is the best way to change the aggressive behavior in a bullying situation. Mediation may be effective in changing behavior of bystanders who are participating in the bullying by egging on the bully, but is not as effective in changing the bully's behavior. This is because the bystanders who are egging on the bully often do not recognize the destructiveness of their behaviors and when an educator approaches them to discuss these behaviors, they tend to be more likely to better understand the damage being done and seek to change their behavior. The MARC (Massachusetts Aggression Reduction Center) has developed a program to help schools better identify and deal with bullying and cyberbullying situations. Their services are free or very low cost and are offered to local schools in Massachusetts in person, and they also offer virtual options and online training programs for educators, parents, students, and health care practitioners. Their program is different than many other bullying programs in that it is an academic center and uses faculty, graduate students, and specially trained undergraduates (who function as role model peers) to incorporate their services at schools and to offer services while helping schools effectively implement the services.

They recommend several steps in an action plan for bullying in schools including the following:

- Discuss the bullying situation with the affected parties and any bystanders
- Inform all involved parties and bystanders about the consequences of bullying
- Offer a Safety and Comfort Plan to the victims (which includes a safe person that they can go to at any time to talk to)
- Inform all appropriate adults (which can include teachers, coaches, bus drivers, guidance counselors, and administrators)
- Develop a plan for less structured locations (such as recess, lunch, library, extracurricular activities, and bus rides to ensure the safety of the victim)
- Follow-up with parents in a timely manner.[30]

All of the US states have laws regarding cyberbullying and criminal charges for violation of these laws, although these laws vary from state to state.[13] Programs in the school systems include social education programs, text-based programs, app-based programs, peer-led counseling programs, and national programs such as Be Safe and Sound in School (B3S) through the National Crime Prevention Council and the US Department of Justice.[11] The fundamental concept of any anti-bullying campaign in the school system or other community group is that there must be defined rules for social encounters and these rules must be practiced and enforced to contribute to a consistently safe environment.[31] Teachers and school personnel need to be appropriately trained to identify cyberbullying and to report to the correct school channels.[13] The US Department of Health and Human Services has an anti-bullying initiative found at Stopbullying.gov (http://www.stopbullying.gov)[32] which contains free educational printable resources. Finally, there are also several other initiatives available for educators including:

- BullyBust (http://www.schoolclimate.org/bullybust)
- Stop Bullying: Speak Up campaign (http://www.cartoonnetwork.com/promos/stopbullying)
- It Gets Better Project (http://www.itgetsbetter.org)
- DoSomething.org (http://www.dosomething.org)
- the Cyberbully Research Center (http://cyberbullying.us)[33]

DISCLOSURE

The authors have no disclosures.

REFERENCES

1. Van Dijck J. The culture of connectivity A critical history of social media. New York: Oxford University Press; 2013.
2. James C, Davis K, Charmaraman L, et al. Digital life and youth well-being, social connectedness, empathy, and narcissism. Pediatrics 2017;140(Suppl 2):S71–5.
3. O'Keeffe G, Clarke-Pearson K, Council on Communications and Media. The impact of social media on children, adolescents and families. Pediatrics 2011; 124:800–4.
4. Valkenburg PM, Peter J. Online communication among adolescents: An integrated model of its attraction, opportunities, and risks. J Adolesc Health 2011; 48:121–7.
5. Moreno MA, Parks MR, Zimmerman FJ, et al. Display of Health Risk Behaviors on MySpace by Adolescents. Prevalence and Associations. Arch Pediatr Adolesc Med 2009;163:27–34.
6. Reid D, Weigle P. Social media use among adolescents: Benefits and risks. Adolesc Psychiatry 2014;4(2):73–80.
7. Fox J, Moreland JJ. The dark side of social networking sites: An exploration of the relational and psychological stressors associated with Facebook use and affordances. Comput Human Behav 2015;45:168–76.
8. Hinduja S, Patchin JW. Bullying, cyberbullying, and suicide. Arch Suicide Res 2010;14:206–21.
9. Konrath S, O'Brien E, Hsing C. Changes in Dispositional Empathy in American College Students Over Time: A Meta-Analysis. Personal Social Psychol Rev 2011;15(2):180–98.
10. Vossen H, Valkenburg P. Do social media foster or curtain adolescents' empathy? A longitudinal study. Comput Human Behav 2016;64:118–24.
11. Waller AP, Lokhande AP, Ekambaram V, et al. Cyberbullying: An Unceasing Threat in Today's Digitalized World. Psychiatr Ann 2018;48(9):408–15.
12. Cyberbullying Research Center. 2020. Available at: cyberbullying.org. Accessed February 8, 2022.
13. Ansary NS. Cyberbullying: Concepts, theories, and correlates informing evidence-based best practices for prevention. Aggression Violent Behav 2020; 50:101343.
14. Glover J, Fritsch SL. KidsAnxiety and Social Media: A Review. Child Adolesc Psychiatr Clin N Am 2018;27:171–82.
15. Eyuboglu M, Eyuboglu D, Pala SC, et al. Traditional school bullying and cyberbullying: Prevalence, the effect on mental health problems and self-harm behavior. Psychiatry Res 2021;297:113730.
16. Van Geel M, Vedder P, Tanilon J. Rela¬tionship between peer victimization, cy-¬berbullying, and suicide in children and adolescents: a meta-analysis. JAMA Pediatr 2014;168(5):435–42.
17. Kann L, McManus T, Harris WA, et al. Youth Risk Behavior Surveillance — United States, 2017. US Department Health Hum Services/Centers Dis Control Prev MMWR 2018;67(8).
18. Reed E, Salazar M, Behar A, et al. Cyber Sexual Harassment: Prevalence and association with substance use, poor mental health, and STI history among sexually active adolescent girls. J Adolescence 2019;75:53–62.
19. Evans-Lacko S, Takizawa R, Brimblecombe N, et al. Childhood bullying victimization is associated with use of mental health services over five decades: a longitudinal nationally representative cohort study. Psychol Med 2017;47:127–35.

20. Hutson E, Melnyk B, Hensley V, et al. Childhood Bullying: Screening and Intervening Practices of Pediatric Primary-care Providers. J Pediatr Health Care November 2019;33(6):E39–45.
21. Strout T, Vessey J, DiFazio R, et al. The Child Adolescent Bullying Scale (CABS): Psychometric evaluation of a new measure. Res Nurs Health 2018;41:252–64.
22. MARC center. Available at: www.MARCcenter.org. Accessed March 14, 2022.
23. Hogan, Strasberger, Twenty Questions and Answers about Media violence and cyberbullying. Pediatr Clin North Am 2020;67:275–91.
24. National Crime Prevention Council. What parents can do about cyberbullying. Available at: https://www.ncpc.org/resources/cyberbullying/what-parents-can-do-about-cyberbullying/. Accessed March 18, 2022.
25. Hinduja S, Patchin JW. Cyberbullying Identification, Prevention, and Response. Cyberbullying Research Center. 2021. Available at: cyberbullying.org. Accessed February 8, 2022.
26. Available at: https://www.healthychildren.org/English/family-life/Media/Pages/How-to-Make-a-Family-Media-Use-Plan.aspx. Accessed April 29, 2022.
27. Available at: http://www.aacap.org/AACAP/Families_and_Youth/Facts_for_Families/FFF-Guide/FFF-Guide-Home.aspx. Accessed April 20, 2022.
28. Rocha S. Talking with teens and families about digital media use. Brown Univ Child Adolesc Behav Lett 2019;35(3):5–7.
29. Ak S, Ozdemir Y, Kuzucu Y, et al. Cybervictimization and cyberbullying: the mediating role of anger, don't anger me! Comput Human Behav 2015;49:437–43.
30. Englander E. Spinning Our Wheels:Improving Our Ability to Respond to Bullying and Cyberbullying. Child Adolesc Psychiatr Clin N Am 2012;21:43–55.
31. Bostic J, Brunt C. Cornered: an Approach to School Bullying and Cyberbullying, and Forensic Implications. Child Adolesc Psychiatr Clin N Am 2011;20:447–65.
32. stopbullying.gov. Available at: http://www.stopbullying.gov. Accessed March 18, 2022.
33. D'Auria J. Cyberbullying Resources for Youth and Their Families. J Pediatr Health Care 2014;28:e19–22.

Mental Health Concerns for College Students

Self-Harm, Suicidal Ideation, and Substance Use Disorders

Brandyn Mason, DO, MME, MHSA

KEYWORDS

• College • Self-harm • Suicidal ideation • Substance use disorder

KEY POINTS

- Prevalence of mental health disorders in college students continues to increase due to the unfamiliar social situations that these individuals are facing for the first time.
- Substance use disorders make up a large amount of these disorders with alcohol use disorder being the most prevalent.
- Suicidal ideations are far more prevalent in college students when compared with same age nonstudents and are even more increased in both racial and sexual minority student groups.
- Socioeconomic, racial, and sexual identity variables also lead to an alteration in the prevalence, severity, and ability to seek mental health assistance in the college student.
- Most college students with mental health disorders do not seek out assistance due to many factors, so identification and treatment of these disorders requires help from the faculty, family, and student body for these individuals.

INTRODUCTION

An increase in the prevalence of all mental illness within college student populations has been demonstrated in a number of different studies. According to the World Health Organization study on the prevalence of mental health issues among college students, 35% of all full-time students studied screened positive for at least one common lifetime mental health disorder and 31% screened positive for at least one of those disorders within the last 12 months before survey completion.[1] These disorders included major depressive disorder, mania/hypomania, generalized anxiety disorder, panic disorder, alcohol use disorder, and drug use disorder with each having a varying degree of correlation to several demographic factors.[1] There are many plausible explanations as to why this increase in mental health disorders among this age group

Carle Foundation Hospital, 611 W Park, Urbana, IL 61802, USA
E-mail address: brandyn.mason@carle.com

Prim Care Clin Office Pract 50 (2023) 47–55
https://doi.org/10.1016/j.pop.2022.10.007
0095-4543/23/© 2022 Elsevier Inc. All rights reserved.

exists, with most agreeing that the major life transition into college with its associated issues of having an unstable life structure leading to feelings of uncertainty and need to explore options while focusing on one's self combine to cause a significant amount of distress in the student's life, all of which increases the likelihood of developing a mental health disorder.[1] In additional to these issues, college students are confronted with adult responsibilities that they most likely have not had before, including financial stability and the development and maintenance of significant relationships.[2] All of these conditions may lead individuals within the college community to place themselves in unfamiliar situations to gain social recognition or to become more insular and avoid fellow students. This leads to more questioning of what the individual is from a metaphysical point of view.

Sociodemographics that correlate the highest with developing both lifetime and 12 months prevalence were female gender, nonheterosexual identification and older age, aged 19 to 20 years or older when beginning college studies.[1] Other demographics that showed some positive correlation were students of unmarried parents, students with at least one deceased parent, those with lower high school rankings (lower 70% of class), extrinsically motivated students and those identifying as having no religious affiliation, although not to the level of previously mentioned demographics.[1] There were no studies that demonstrated having more than one of these correlates actually infers an additive risk to the development of mental health problems in this age group. These mental disorders could also create life-long implications due to the double risk of college discontinuation without receiving a degree, which is consistent with approximately 20% of students with mental disorders identifying its negative impact on their academic performance and demonstrated by an average decrease of 0.2 to 0.3 grade point average (GPA) on diagnosis of a mental health disorder.[3] These life-long implications could be furthered observed by an "increase in physical and emotional problems in the mid to long term, labor market marginalization, worse quality of sleep, and dysfunctional relationships" with those with mental health diagnosis at the college age.[4] These issues could then create the unstable mentality for the students allowing them to be prone to increasing stressors that lead to more mental disorders and a cycle of worsening mental stability.

Substance Use Disorders

Substance use disorders are a large part of mental disorders within the college student population with alcohol use disorder being the most prevalent of the group. According to Wagstaff and Welfare, approximately 65% of college students have ingested alcohol within any given month and 44% of the college population meet criteria for binge drinking, which was even more prevalent during the first semester of college, with 50% of men and 33% of women ingesting at levels 2 to 3 times the binge drinking rate during this time period.[5] Being enrolled in college also affects alcohol consumption, where college students not only consume a greater quantity but also suffer from more alcohol-related consequences when compared with their same age noncollege peers.[6] Hazardous drinking has been documented in various prevalence rates (33% to 57%) in American college students and is defined as "a large intake of alcohol that increases one's risk of alcohol-related problems/consequences."[6] In the study by Paulus and Zvolensky, it was identified that more than three-quarters of the students who were studied demonstrated at least moderate drinking and that same study group showed nearly 60% of these individuals had elevated anxiety sensitivity scores, defined as a fear of anxiety-related bodily sensations.[6] When these numbers are examined closer, it demonstrates that those identified as hazardous drinkers showed a 77.5% elevated anxiety sensitivity demonstrating an association with hazardous drinking and anxiety sensitivity.[6] This also demonstrates that there is a possiblecorrelation between hazardous drinking and other mental health diagnosis.

Alcohol use disorders can also co-occur with gambling disorders because they are both manifestations of risk-taking behavior.[7] College students are susceptible to these due to their elevated rate of impulsivity and the earlier onset of these disorders the greater the risk of increasing impulsivity to continue long term.[7] So if developed during the freshman years, which was previously identified as a high alcohol ingestion period, the likelihood of having lifetime impulsivity-related problems greatly increases. Individuals with these co-occurring disease states have demonstrated poorer health outcome behaviors, including tobacco use, and partaking in health risk behaviors, including decreased seatbelt use and increased driving under the influence.[7] Because heavy alcohol use may exacerbate negative thoughts and depressive symptoms and the association with suicidal thoughts and ideations, alcohol use disorder has an association with suicidal ideation and behavior among university students.[8]

Motivational interviewing and feedback given on a personal level has been demonstrated to be the most effective interventions for college students with alcohol use disorders.[9] The need for improved coping skills due to the effect of negative effect on amount of alcohol consumption allows for sustainability of the intervention on reduced alcohol consumption in the future.[9] This could be accomplished by using mindfulness to help individuals become more aware of the affective states and reduce impulsivity without increasing the need for those same individuals to engage in substance misuse.[9] Instructing students on being more open and mindful of themselves and their current state has a more profound effect on long-term success of treatment and decreasing the prevalence of alcohol use disorder both in this population and those post college age.

Nonmedical prescription opioid (NMPO) use has a suggested prevalence of approximately 10% in the college student community, although studies have demonstrated varying rates from 7.5% to 32% across separate samples.[10] There are several factors that increase the likelihood of NMPO use but those that have been demonstrated to have the highest correlation are "physical pain, anxiety, depression, executive functioning deficits, and other comorbid substance misuse" with suicidal and depressive feelings being the primary motivated independent of physical pain presence.[10] This can be demonstrated by 56% of those college students using NMPO recreationally also meeting the criteria for major depressive disorder.[10] A usual pathway to NMPO use is by the need to decrease the subjective pain that they experience and believing that these medication cure all types of pain, regardless of whether they are physical, emotional, or spiritual manifestations of the pain.

Suicidal Ideations: Prevalence, Risks, and Screening

There is a drastic difference in the prevalence of suicidal ideation, 24% vs 9%, and attempts, 9% vs 2.7%, in the college students when compared with the adult population as a whole.[11] There are several factors that predispose students to suicidal ideations and attempts that include "depression, impulsivity, poverty, poor neighborhood, lack of parental warmth, and/or abuse and family conflict" along with anxiety, poor self-esteem, and substance use.[12] Another important contributing factor is those that identify as a sexual minority, that is, lesbian, gay, or bisexual, even though these groups tend to use offered mental health at a greater rate than those that identify as heterosexual.[11] These patients, who often inhabit marginalized identities, demonstrated a double or triple increase in the rates of suicidal ideations, with those identifying as bisexual having the highest increases, likely due to the difficulty navigating 2 different social circles, the heterosexual and homosexual groups, while not fully having a sense of belonging.[11] Understanding the predeposition to suicidal ideations in these vulnerable patients may help identify disorders earlier and prevent some suicidal attempts.

Under-represented students have a similar path, including a significantly lower utilization of offered mental health services, which may in turn lead to underdiagnosis of mental health disease states in these also vulnerable populations.[11] Although under-represented patients, identified as Hispanics, Blacks, and Asians, showed significantly decreased rates of diagnosis of anxiety, depression, combined anxiety and depression, or other diagnosis, the rate of suicidality or self-injurious behavior were not as pronounced.[11] Some of the decreased utilization may be correlated with cultural factors that include the stigma of mental health disease in certain ethnic populations or the inability to recognize mental health problems within the individual due to this same stigma.[11] Studies have demonstrated that the Black community finds mental illness as a weakness and because of such, standardized instruments for detecting mental illness may not be as sensitive in these populations.[11]

Emotional dysregulation and partaking in self-damaging behaviors have demonstrated an increase in suicide risk among college students where emotional dysregulation is defined as encompassing "non-acceptance of emotional responses, difficulties engaging in goal-directed behavior, impulse control difficulties, lack of emotional awareness, limited access to emotion regulation strategies and lack of emotional clarity" both as individual components and to a higher extent when in combination.[12] The view of oneself being burdensome to others along with the lack of perceived meaningful relationships is an important concept within emotional dysregulation and leads to continued painful or dangerous experience engagement and eventually the ability of the student to commit suicide.[12] Self-damaging behaviors include several concepts including those with potential to cause physical harm to self, nonsuicidal self-injury, and substance use disorders.[12] Self-damaging behaviors in the college student generally manifest as substance misuse, physical altercations with others, and lack of common safety concerns and precautions.[12] Although these self-damaging behaviors may lead to increased suicide risk, the main purpose of these events to the student is to assist in relieving or reducing their negative emotions.[12]

Attention deficit hyperactivity disorder (ADHD) is a commonly occurring mental health condition in the college student that also often creates a decreased ability to adjust to college life resulting in decreased academic achievement, reduction in relationships that are meaningful, and an overall lower quality of life.[13] Due to these social issues, first-year college students have a significantly elevated prevalence, up to 4 times as high, of suicidal ideations and attempts when compared with those students not diagnosed with ADHD.[13] Depression co-occurs in ADHD students at an approximate rate of 32.3%, which also furthers the risk of suicidality in this patient population.

Suicidality in the college student is a growing concern and many studies have demonstrated that before a student's death by suicide about 50% visited a primary care provider within the month preceding and 25% had been under the care of a mental health professional the month preceding the event.[14] The need to develop a better tool to screen for suicide risk in the college student in order to decrease the loss of life is paramount. According to Frick, Butler and deBoer, there was a slightly higher prevalence of suicidality during the sophomore year when compared with all other years, which were equivalent (**Table 1**).[14] That same study identified that increased awareness and universal screening of college students demonstrated a significant increase in referrals to the mental health provider along with more than doubling the number of individuals that scheduled appointments with these providers.[14]

Table 1	
Suicide risk during academic year	
College Year	Positively Screened for Suicide (%)
Freshman	11.58
Sophomore	17.68
Junior	11.88
Senior	10.87

Early life suicidal thoughts and behaviors is a common occurrence before entering college, with approximately one-third of college students having these thoughts or behaviors before enrollment, which can lead to poorer academic performance, increased college dropout rate, and persistent mental and physical problems.[15] Several adverse childhood events could increase the risk of suicidality in college students but none seems to be higher than those that experience childhood abuse, with about a 2.5 times higher prevalence, and even a higher risk for those who experienced sexual abuse and complex abuse.[15] Recent studies also demonstrate that there seems to be a ceiling effect to the "impact of childhood adversities and related toxic stress" on the risk of future suicidal thoughts and behaviors.[15]

Special Populations

There are many demographical variables that influence the mental health of a college student, which include gender, sexual identity, ethnicity, place of origin, and involvement in collegiate athletics. Each of these demographics changes the perceived need for counseling services and mental health diagnosis in these groups, whereas being female or sexual minorities increased the perceived need of services and being male, from lower socioeconomic backgrounds, or an international student decreased the perceived need for mental health services.[16]

When compared with heterosexual peers, individuals that indentify as lesbian, gay, bisexual, queer, or trans (LGBQT +) demonstrate higher prevalence of anxiety and depression symptoms, including hopelessness and feeling overwhelmed.[17] A review of college mental health services found that only about 30% of campuses mention individual services for these individuals and only 5% of those same campuses have support groups for the LGBQT + community.[17] With the perceived need for increased mental health services in this group, LGBQT + individuals were 105% more likely to receive treatment of anxiety, 206% more likely to receive treatment of depression, 194% more likely to see a mental health therapist, and 93% more likely to seek out mental health care from the college's offered services.[17]

Research has demonstrated that college students identifying as Black have a greater perceived social stigma with mental health and negative opinions toward seeking assistance with mental health issues when identified leading to the usage of about half of the mental health services that their white peers use.[18] The history of struggle is a culturally accepted normality that leads to the need for increased endurance when compared with other social groups, which may explain the decreased pursuing of services for treatment and diagnosis.[18] This lack of drive to seek mental health assistance also leads to an increased risk of suicidality where 17% of black college students screen positive for suicide risk and only one-third of those individuals seek any mental health services.[18] Lifetime rates of discrimination (**Table 2**) differ by ethnic groups but its elevated rates lead to perceived discrimination

Table 2	
Racial discrimination risk for self-identified racial groups	
Ethnic Group	Lifetime Risk of Racial Discrimination in the United States (%)
Black	75
Pacific Islander	71
Asian	60
American Indian	55
Hispanic	50

creating many mental health problems and outcomes and are influenced mostly by who the offender was.[19]

Social stigma toward mental health is also a strong part of the culture of college athletes leading to an underutilization of services and decrease in seeking a mental health diagnosis.[20] When comparing male and female athletes to each other, there was no difference in mental health outcomes, energy levels, sexual regret, or alcohol consumption but there was an increase in drug usage and aggressive behavior in male athletes.[20] An increase in alcohol consumption was correlated with improved psychological outcomes in the female athletes only, which was presumed to be a cause of improved social connectedness.[20] Mental health was most likely underdiagnosed but what was observed is that male athletes tended to fit hypermasculine roles of aggression and female athletes turned to social drinking as a way to correct their psychological stressors.

International students have an increased risk of developing mental health problems due to the additional risk factors that they face, including language barriers, culture shock, and changes to normal learning and living environments.[21] Due to similar culture views on mental health as the black college community, these individuals are also less likely to seek care from mental health providers, which may lead to a false reduction in the prevalence of mental health disease in these individuals.[21] International students were found to have equivocal rates of depression and decreased rates of anxiety and suicidal ideation when compared with domestic students but had a significantly increased rate of suicidal attempts.[21]

Type of college, community versus 4-year University, also have a significant effect on mental health. The student population of community colleges differs by having a higher proportion of nonwhite students, those that come from lower socioeconomic backgrounds, and students who are employed full-time during their schooling the cohort also tends to be older as well.[22] When indicating the most likely stressor leading to the development of mental health disorders, financial stress and stability was indicated as the cause with 70.4% of students enrolled in community college indicating that their financial situation was always stressful.[22] This financial stressor also led to decreased academic performance and increased dropout rates without earning a degree.[22]

Treatment and next Steps

The students that seek mental health services through their college campuses showed a mixed amount of disease states, with 51% diagnosed with anxiety 41% diagnosed with depression and 34% dealing with relationship issues and 24.5% being prescribed psychotropic medications.[23] The difficult nature with college campus mental health assistance is that most of the individuals that receive care in these clinics are self-referred and not screened for mental health by any official means. The feeling of belonging and a good foundation of social support has been demonstrated to reduce the sense of burden to others and decrease the likelihood of engaging in suicidal behaviors due to the increased sense of connectedness to others.[24]

Due to college students initially reaching out through personal relationships, friends and family, first before seeking other avenues for mental health care, the need for mental health first aid may improve outcomes if adapted more widely.[25] "Mental health first aid, which was initially developed and implemented in Australia, is a standardized program that trains people how to support others and provide initial help during mental health crisis situations."[25] This program, which entails formal training of length that can vary from 8 to 13 hours, has been found to improve students' knowledge about mental health and increase the effectiveness of the treatment, if sought, while improving the confidence in students to offer aid during mental health crisis and direct fellow students to available resources.[25]

Online therapy has been an increasingly used option during COVID-19 pandemic and has varying benefits in the development of therapeutic relationship. Studies have shown that online therapy does assist in some of the initial difficulties with direct interpersonal contact, as these events can be intimidating because the patient feels like they are being judged and analyzed by an individual they have not previously met leading to difficulty with clear and appropriate communication.[26] Once the initial therapeutic relationship is developed, online therapy begins to lose its effectiveness because questions about security and confidentiality of the information come into effect.[26]

When developing an effective student mental health service line on campus there are several factors that will improve the success of the offered services: involving students and peers, matching capacity with clinic services demands, the use of informational technology, being as visible as possible, modeling vulnerability and self-care by the treatment teams, adaptability of offered services and building a team that promotes collegiality.[27] Using peers and students that have dealt with mental health issues and asking these individuals to promote and discuss these issues among the campus community can provide a significant benefit to the overall mental health of the community.[27] The use of information technology will vary by student but having a multitude of different options for communication allows more individuals to seek and obtain the care that they may need.[27] Many campus mental health clinics have a wait list, approximately 44%, which would indicate to make sure that more services than what can be provided are not offered to the community.[27] Not all students need a required timetable for services but rather would require the ability to adjust the need based on social events, academic requirements, and interpersonal relationships.[27] Mental health care does increase the risk of burnout among those providers and does require a collegial environment to seek help among each other to ensure that the care provided to the students is still of the highest quality.[27]

CLINICS CARE POINTS

- College students undergo great social transformation that makes them more susceptible to mental health disease.
- College students have increased impulsivity that increased their risk of substance abuse disorders and may manifest as increased risky health behaviors such as decreased seat belt wearing or increased tobacco use.
- Racial minorities seek out mental health services at a significantly decreased rate and should be screened often for mental health illness alone because they are unlikely to share with family present.

- Gear mental health services for LGBQT + individuals toward those that are more familiar with best-practices for the treatment of patients who inhabit those identities because they often do not have the same stressors as their heterosexual counterparts.
- Consider the use of mental health first aid and the factors that make up an effective student mental health program when developing screening and treatment protocols for this group.

DISCLOSURE

Brandyn Mason has no financial or commercial conflicts of interest and receives no funding for the completion of this article.

ACKNOWLEDGMENTS

Carle Health (Employer), Frances Drone-Silvers (Medical Librian for Carle Health), Rachel Trimble (Wife, for being my constant source of support).

REFERENCES

1. Auerbach RP, Mortier P, Bruffaerts R, et al. 19.1 World Health Organization World Mental Health Surveys International College Student Project (WMH-ICS): Prevalence and Distribution of Mental Disorders. J Am Acad Child Adolesc Psychiatry 2018;57(10):S297.
2. Pedrelli P. College Students: Mental Health Problems and Treatment Considerations. Acad Psychiatry 2014;39(5):503–11.
3. Bruffaerts R, Mortier P, Kiekens G, et al. Mental health problems in college freshmen: Prevalence and academic functioning. J Affective Disord 2018;225: 97–103.
4. Ramón-Arbués E, Gea-Caballero V, Granada-López JM, et al. The Prevalence of Depression, Anxiety and Stress and Their Associated Factors in College Students. Int J Environ Res Public Health 2020;17(19):7001.
5. Wagstaff JF, Welfare LE. Brief Alcohol Screening and Intervention for College Students on Campus: Lessons From Experienced Practitioners. J Coll Couns 2021; 24(2):115–31.
6. Paulus DJ, Zvolensky MJ. The prevalence and impact of elevated anxiety sensitivity among hazardous drinking college students. Drug Alcohol Depend 2020; 209:107922.
7. King SM, Whelan JP. Gambling and Alcohol Problems during the College Years: Personality, Physical and Emotional Health and Gambling Beliefs. Issues Ment Health Nurs 2020;41(12):1095–103.
8. Coryell W, Horwitz A, Albucher R, et al. Alcohol intake in relation to suicidal ideation and behavior among university students. J Am Coll Health 2021;1–5. https://doi.org/10.1080/07448481.2021.1950160.
9. Cotter EW, Hawthorne DJ, Gerker C, et al. A Pilot Mindfulness Intervention to Reduce Heavy Episodic Drinking. J Coll Couns 2021;24(2):178–92.
10. Weyandt LL, Gudmundsdottir BG, Shepard E, et al. Nonmedical Prescription Opioid Use among a Sample of College Students: Prevalence and Predictors. Pharmacy 2021;9(2):106.
11. Liu CH, Stevens C, Wong SHM, et al. The prevalence and predictors of mental health diagnoses and suicide among U.S. college students: Implications for addressing disparities in service use. Depress Anxiety 2018;36(1):8–17.

12. Owusu-Ansah FE, Addae AA, Peasah BO, et al. Suicide among university students: prevalence, risks and protective factors. Health Psychol Behav Med 2020;8(1):220–33.
13. Haliczer LA, Harnedy LE, Oakley M, et al. Clarifying the Role of Multiple Self-Damaging Behaviors in the Association Between Emotion Dysregulation and Suicide Risk Among College Students. J Prim Prev 2021;42(5):473–92.
14. Eddy LD, Eadeh HM, Breaux R, et al. Prevalence and predictors of suicidal ideation, plan, and attempts, in first-year college students with ADHD. J Am Coll Health 2019;68(3):313–9.
15. Frick MG, Butler SA, deBoer DS. Universal suicide screening in college primary care. J Am Coll Health 2019;1–6. https://doi.org/10.1080/07448481.2019.1645677.
16. Husky MM, Sadikova E, Lee S, et al. Childhood adversities and mental disorders in first-year college students: results from the World Mental Health International College Student Initiative. Psychol Med 2022;1–11. https://doi.org/10.1017/s0033291721004980.
17. Seehuus M, Moeller RW, Peisch V. Gender effects on mental health symptoms and treatment in college students. J Am Coll Health 2019;1–8. https://doi.org/10.1080/07448481.2019.1656217.
18. Bourdon JL, Liadis A, Tingle KM, et al. Trends in mental health service utilization among LGB+ college students. J Am Coll Health 2020;1–9. https://doi.org/10.1080/07448481.2019.1706537.
19. Busby DR, Zheng K, Eisenberg D, et al. Black college students at elevated risk for suicide: Barriers to mental health service utilization. J Am Coll Health 2019;1–7. https://doi.org/10.1080/07448481.2019.1674316.
20. de Souza NL, Esopenko C, Conway FN, et al. Patterns of health behaviors affecting mental health in collegiate athletes. J Am Coll Health 2019;1–8. https://doi.org/10.1080/07448481.2019.1682591.
21. Yeung TS, Hyun S, Zhang E, et al. Prevalence and correlates of mental health symptoms and disorders among US international college students. J Am Coll Health 2021;1–7. https://doi.org/10.1080/07448481.2020.1865980.
22. Lipson SK, Phillips MV, Winquist N, et al. Mental Health Conditions Among Community College Students: A National Study of Prevalence and Use of Treatment Services. Psychiatr Serv 2021;(appi.ps):2020004. https://doi.org/10.1176/appi.ps.202000437.
23. Forbes FJM, Whisenhunt BL, Citterio C, et al. Making mental health a priority on college campuses: implementing large scale screening and follow-up in a high enrollment gateway course. J Am Coll Health 2019;1–8. https://doi.org/10.1080/07448481.2019.1665051.
24. Restrepo DM, Spokas M. Social support moderates the relationship between interpersonal trauma and suicidal behaviors among college students. J Am Coll Health 2021;1–7. https://doi.org/10.1080/07448481.2021.1967961.
25. Liang M, Chen Q, Guo J, et al. Mental health first aid improves mental health literacy among college students: A meta-analysis. J Am Coll Health 2021;1–10. https://doi.org/10.1080/07448481.2021.1925286.
26. Hanley T, Wyatt C. A systematic review of higher education students' experiences of engaging with online therapy. Counselling Psychotherapy Res 2020. https://doi.org/10.1002/capr.12371.
27. Davis RA, Wolfe J, Heiman N. Increasing utilization of student mental health services on a college campus: Eight actionable tips. J Am Coll Health 2021;1–5. https://doi.org/10.1080/07448481.2021.1909035.

Health Disparities, Substance-Use Disorders, and Primary-Care

Angela L. Colistra, PhD, LPC, CAADC, CCS[a,b,*], Andrea Ward, DO[a,c],
Erin Smith, DO[a,b,d]

KEYWORDS

- Primary-care ● Addiction ● Disparity ● Drug policy ● Inequity ● Social determinants
- Treatment ● Health care disparities

KEY POINTS

- Stigma remains the largest health disparity of treating substance-use disorder in primary-care yet to be overcome.
- Educational models that consider the role of stigma in medical and behavioral health training are needed to push care forward.
- System and payer challenges need continued considerations for interdisciplinary care teams to be valued within primary-care.

INTRODUCTION

Treating people with substance-use disorders (SUD) throughout history has been plagued with disparate conditions inside and outside of the primary-care settings. Some challenges include:

- The stigma associated with substance-use disorders alone makes it a condition that people struggle to accept as a disease that warrants treatment whether it be medical, behavioral, or spiritual care.
- Addiction is more likely to be viewed as a moral failing that requires grit, determination, and "tough love" to overcome its grips than it is to be seen as a disease with available medical, behavioral, and spiritual treatment and support pathways.
- The local news portrays weak, dirty, criminal individuals who fall victim to substance-use disorder (SUD) and this alone makes it less likely that individuals

[a] Lehigh Valley Health Network Department of Family Medicine, 707 Hamilton Street, 8th Floor, Allentown, PA 18101, USA; [b] University of South Florida Morsani College of Medicine, Tampa, FL, USA; [c] LVPG Family Medicine-Hamburg, Lehigh Valley Health Network, 700 Hawk Ridge Drive, Hamburg, PA 19526, USA; [d] Neighborhood Centers of the Lehigh Valley, 218 North 2nd Street, Allentown, PA 18102, USA
* Corresponding author.
E-mail address: angela.colistra@lvhn.org

Prim Care Clin Office Pract 50 (2023) 57–69
https://doi.org/10.1016/j.pop.2022.11.001
0095-4543/23/Published by Elsevier Inc.

will accept their diagnosis or the recommended treatment to avoid this social stigma.
- Lack of awareness about or trust in the systems that provide the medical and behavioral treatments that treat the symptoms of SUD makes it less likely people will accept these as a valid option for their healing.

These barriers illustrate that *stigma* is the largest health disparity in treating SUD in primary-care yet to be overcome.

The same is true for primary-care providers who decide to heal substance-use disorders; the stigma continues to often pervade the medical profession, thus making it difficult to understand the readiness of primary-care as a specialty to show up for this call to action. There is no doubt we see more primary-care doctors willing to provide care. However, many systemic and social determinants of health make it challenging for primary-care providers to heed the call to action due to the system barriers that make it difficult for these providers to stay healthy while providing this care.

Some major barriers within the system include a lack of alignment between health care systems and payers, illustrating that they value this care by providing appropriate time structures for patient encounters, compensation, and resource allocation for the primary-care interdisciplinary treatment team members. The current climate is fraught with challenges and opportunities to recognize that treating people with SUDs can be both primary-care and specialty care.

Primary-care acknowledging that SUDs are independent, chronic conditions will require continued paradigm shifts within health care systems and communities in the coming decade which can then lead to restored healing for patients by treating them through a true multi-disciplinary approach. Once the willingness of primary-care providers (medical and behavioral) and the value given to these providers by the health care system and payers aligns together, it can unlock a wave of healing just by reducing this one health care disparity: access to care.

This article reviews the history, definitions, and background knowledge that has brought us to this point of time in understanding the history of treating patients with SUDs in primary-care and the related health disparities. We also leave you with clinical care points to consider when treating patients with substance-use disorders in primary-care.

History

How we arrived at where primary-care offices are today in the journey of treating SUDs involves reflecting on how we currently provide medical and some behavioral health care for other substance-use disorders, including alcohol-use disorder, tobacco use disorder, and the rising frequency of the need to be familiar with treatment protocols for methamphetamine use disorder.[1] In addition, we see more discussion on Office Based Opioid Treatment[2] than in years prior. One major consideration influencing how care is diagnosed ultimately impacts treatment availability.

- The American Psychological Association's Diagnostic and Statistical Manual (DSM) of Mental Disorders, edition 1 in 1952 identified "addiction" as part of sociopathic mind disturbance.[3]
- In subsequent iterations, addictions were placed alongside personality disorders and eventually morphed into an umbrella description of "substance-use disorder" that later included subcategories within addiction.[4]
- Although the definition of substance-use disorder is now classified as a "primary mental health disorder," before revised iterations of the DSM manual in the 1980s, substance-use disorders were conceptualized as manifestations of

underlying primary psychopathology, incurring a large paradigm shift that occurred in about half a century.[5]

This shift in thinking helps to lay the groundwork to address and treat substance-use disorders via a holistic approach in primary-care while understanding the complex relationship among pathology, personal circumstance, cultural influence, and bias when supporting this population. Substance-use disorder treatment originally involved the patient under the care of a multidisciplinary team consisting of behavioral health and consultants with specific training in addiction medicine/substance-use disorders and was outside the scope of primary-care. These models align with the American Society of Addiction Medicine (ASAM) Criteria which are the most widely used guidelines for placement, continued stay, transfer, or discharge of patients with addiction and co-occurring conditions and provide the following placement decisions:[6]

- Prevention/early intervention
- Outpatient
- Intensive outpatient/partial hospitalization
- Residential/inpatient
- Intensive inpatient

In addition to the DSM and the ASAM Criteria, SUD treatment in primary-care evolved when several entities came together; some of these major shifts have included:

- The expansion of behavioral health into primary-care, including when the concept of substance-use disorder as a chronic disease was realized and the recognition of the high likelihood of a history of trauma (physical, psychological, or both) co-occurring in patients with SUD.
- The creation of the patient-centered medical home model
- An expansion of co-located care management in the primary-care setting
- The schedule III recommendation for buprenorphine made in 2002 by the Department of Health and Human Services (among other changes)[7–12] (**Table 1**).

The missions of primary-care and treating substance-use disorders are similar: both require compassionate, goal-oriented, cost-effective care with the establishment of long-standing patient-provider relationships focusing on the development of trust and overall wellness. Substance-use disorder treatment requires compassionate providers who can relationship-build with the goal of continuity of care throughout the treatment course.

One of the benefits of treating substance-use disorders within primary-care settings is that patients can receive treatment of their substance-use disorders by receiving available medications to help curb cravings or manage withdrawals while also gaining coordination of and ideally access to behavioral health services. This ability to reduce barriers and improve access to what is relatively complex care is needed to get more people the care they need in a timely fashion (**Table 2**).

The language we use to discuss SUDs and their relevant treatments perhaps has become one of the most important discussions of this decade. The publication of *Addictionary*[17] which provides a complete list of language often associated with SUDs, includes the use of a "stigma alert" for harmful terms while recommending alternative words for replacement. This simple yet profound tool can be used as a tool to further destigmatize our care while moving towards a unified language that promotes health and healing. See **Table 3**.

Table 1 Important dates: substance-use disorder treatment in America	
~10,000BCE	Substance-use disorder/addiction diagnosis follows a convoluted and complicated course throughout history. Humans have used mind-altering substances for different reasons presumably dating back to 10,000BCE, with medical and nonmedical intentions for use.[5]
1700s	Addiction medicine, or the study and treatment of addictive diseases, has developed over the last few hundred years in America. Specifically, "alcoholism" was named as a disease in America in the early 1700s by Benjamin Rush, a medical doctor, and a signer of the Declaration of Independence.[13]
1930s	Alcoholism wasn't considered a disease until the 1930s when Bill Wilson and Dr Bob Smith founded "Alcoholics Anonymous" (AA). Both individuals seeking recovery from alcoholism, and through this, the concept of alcoholism as a disease spread throughout the United States and world.[13]
1950	In the early 1950s, the modern addiction medicine movement began with the formation of the New York Medical Society on Alcoholism and its recognition of alcoholism as a disease. Not long after in California, Narcotics Anonymous (NA) was formed, as Alcoholics Anonymous specifically excluded substances other than alcohol from its scope.[13]
1960	The drug revolution in America in the 1960s led to another paradigm shift of understanding that treatments for addiction were imperative. Its medicalization allowed health care professionals to view addiction or substance-use disorder as a disease, opening up future channels for its treatment as a chronic disease.[13]
1970	On the heels of the Vietnam war with growing substance-use disorders among returning war veterans, the Nixon administration formed the Special Action Office of Drug Abuse Prevention (SAODP) followed by the National Institute of Drug Abuse (NIDA) and the National Institute of Alcoholism and Alcohol Abuse (NIAA). These agencies allowed for funding available for substance-use disorder treatment.[13]
1980	Various medical societies organized to eventually form The American Society of Addiction Medicine and eventually created a certification program. The ASAM placement criteria, the most widely used criteria for treatment decision placement began work toward their 1st iteration of the placement criteria.[14]
1990	In 1990, the American Medical Association House of Delegates acknowledged "Addiction Medicine" as a medical specialty.[13]
2000	In 2000, the Drug Abuse Treatment Act authorized the use of schedule III drugs such as buprenorphine and naloxone in the treatment of opioid addiction by qualified physicians in a medical setting.[13,15]
2009	The integration of board certification in Addiction Medicine beginning in 2009 integration of behavioral health services in substance-use disorder treatment, and the ongoing research supporting substance-use disorder/addiction as a chronic, treatable disease have continued to pave the way for integration into the health care system today
2021	The US Department of Health and Human Services updated The Practice Guidelines for the Administration of Buprenorphine for Treating Opioid-use Disorder. Physicians in certain states without a waiver can use this exemption will be limited to treating no more than 30 patients with buprenorphine for opioid-use disorder at any one time (note: the 30-patient cap does not apply to hospital-based physicians, such as Emergency Department physicians).[16]

Table 2
Medications used to treat substance-use disorders in primary-care

Medications Used to Treat Substance-Use Disorders	
Opioid-use disorder	*Alcohol-use disorder*
Buprenorphine (oral, subcutaneous injection)	Acamprosate (oral)
Naltrexone (intramuscular injection)	Naltrexone (intramuscular injection)
Methadone (oral)	Disulfuram (oral)
Opioid overdose prevention medication	
Naloxone (nasal inhalation)	

Data from Chanell Baylor. Medication-Assisted treatment (MAT) | SAMHSA - Substance Abuse and Mental Health Services Administration. Samhsa.gov. Published 2021. https://www.samhsa.gov/medication-assisted-treatment.

Although the language remains essential, we must also recognize the sheer amount of people who have been diagnosed with a substance-use disorder makes it necessary that we expand care.

The staggering number of people who have used and who later go on to develop SUD speaks to the need for expanded care. Of the number of people aged 12 or older in the United States in 2020, 58.7% (or 162 million people) used tobacco, alcohol, or an illicit drug in the last month. This is also defined as 'current use', including 50% (or 138.5 million people) who drank alcohol, 18.7% (or 51.7mllion people) who used a tobacco product, and 13.5% (or 37.3 million people) who used an illicit drug.[33] In 2020, 40.3 million people aged 12 or older (or 14.5%) had a SUD in the past year, including 28.3 million who had alcohol-use disorder, 18.4 million who had an illicit drug use disorder, and 6.5 million people who had both alcohol and illicit drug use disorder.[33] Despite the obvious need, of these individuals only a small fraction were able to access appropriate care. Hence, the aim of SUD treatment in primary-care is to make it easier for people to access care by meeting the patient where they with the appropriate evidenced-based medical and behavioral treatment in a cost-effective and timely manner.

Background

Owing to the nature of substance-use disorder and the progressively detrimental decline in overall health of the individuals affected by addiction, in addition to existing societal structures, the treatment of this condition is further challenged by many concurrent health disparities. Although SUD treatment exists throughout primary-care offices offering Medicated Assisted Treatment (MAT), in addition to the incorporation of behavioral health approaches and utilization of rehabilitation facilities, many people afflicted by SUD find that access to care is a limitation to treatment. Whether these disparities be transportation access, lack of resources in rural areas, the influences of systemic racism, poor support for treatment regionally, legal implications of substance-use, or access to even the basics of health care, many prospective SUD patients find significant obstacles to obtaining appropriate care for their illness (**Fig. 1** for a more complete list of barriers). Current literature supports the working development of methods to overcome these limitations, but as drug use continues to serve a major impact on communities and families everywhere, further research and planning for overcoming health inequities is needed.[34,35]

Methods to improve treatment successes related to health disparities are being examined closely to improve the care of this vulnerable population. Many studies

Table 3
Keywords and definitions

Definitions	
Preventable differences in the burden of disease, injury, violence, or opportunities to achieve optimal health that are experienced by socially disadvantaged populations.[19]	Health/health care disparities
A treatable, chronic medical disease involving complex interactions among brain circuits, genetics, the environment, and an individual's life experiences.[20]	Addiction
As defined by the American Academy of Family Physicians, primary-care is the provision of integrated, accessible health care services by physicians and the health care teams who are accountable for addressing a large majority of personal health care needs, developing a sustained partnership with patients, and practicing in the context of family and community. The care is person-centered, team-based, community aligned, and designed to achieve better health, better care, and lower costs.[21] The World Health Organization (WHO) acknowledges primary-care as a reinterpreted concept since 1978, redeveloped to facilitate the coordination of future primary health care efforts at the global, national, and local levels. The WHO defines primary-care as "a whole-of society-approach to health that aims at ensuring the highest possible level of health and well-being and their equitable distribution by focusing on people's needs and as early as possible along the continuum from health promotion and disease prevention to treatment, rehabilitation and palliative care, and close as feasible to people's everyday environment."[22]	Primary-care
An umbrella term for care that addresses any behavioral problems bearing on health, including mental health and substance abuse conditions, stress-linked physical symptoms, patient activation and health behaviors. There are many health care settings and performed by many clinicians and health coaches of various disciplines or training.[23]	Behavioral health care
The medical home model is a method intended to improve health care in America by transforming how primary-care is delivered and organized. The Agency for Healthcare Research and Quality (AHRQ) defines a medical home as a model of the organization of primary-care that delivers the core functions of primary health care, encompassing the following five attributes: (1) comprehensive care, (2) patient-centered, (3) coordinated care, (4) accessible services, (5) quality and safety.[24]	Patient-centered medical home
A model of health care delivery that strives to meet patient needs and preferences by actively engaging patients as full participants in their care while encouraging and supporting all health care	Team-based care

(*continued on next page*)

Table 3	
(continued)	
Definitions	
professionals to function to the full extent of their education, certification, and licensure. The health care team includes two or more health care professionals who work collaboratively with patients and their caregivers to accomplish shared goals. Teams can involve a wide range of team members in a variety of health care settings.[25]	
Conditions in the environments where people are born, live, work, play, worship, and age that affect a wide range of health, functioning, and quality of life. Five larger domains include economic stability, education access and quality, health care access and quality, neighborhood and built environment, and social and community context.[26]	Social determinants of health
An approach to the delivery of behavioral health services that includes awareness of the impact it can have across settings, services, and populations; it views trauma through an ecological and cultural lens and recognizes that context plays a significant role in how individuals perceive and process traumatic events, whether acute or chronic. TIC involves vigilance in anticipating and avoiding institutional processes and individual practices that are likely to retraumatize individuals who already have histories of trauma.[27]	Trauma informed care
Defined by the American Psychological Association as the negative social attitude attached to a characteristic of an individual that may be regarded as a mental, physical, or social deficiency. A stigma implies social disapproval and can lead unfairly to discrimination against and exclusion of the individual.[28]	Stigma
Unconscious mental processes that lead to associations and reactions that are automatic and without intention; actors have no awareness of the associations with a stimulus.[29]	Implicit bias
Form of bias that includes preferences, beliefs, and attitudes of which people are generally consciously aware, personally endorse, and can identify and communicate.[29]	Explicit bias
Defined by the Pennsylvania Department of Health and Human Services, "COEs" were established to provide care management services to individuals with opioid-use disorder. They consist of a multidisciplinary group of individuals including case managers, social workers, certified recovery specialists, physicians, tailored to meet the needs of the recovery community.[30]	Centers of excellence
Substance Abuse and Mental Health Services Administration is an agency within the US Department of Health and Human Services that leads	SAMHSA

(continued on next page)

Table 3 (*continued*)	
Definitions	
public health efforts to advance behavioral health of the nation. Their mission is to reduce the impact of substance abuse and mental illness on America's communities.[31]	
A professional medical society founded in 1954 that represents physicians, clinicians and other associated professionals in the field of addiction medicine. ASAM is dedicated to increasing access and improving the quality of addiction treatment, educating physicians and the public, supporting research and prevention, and promoting the appropriate role of physicians in the care of patients with addiction.[32]	ASAM
The use of medications in combination with counseling and behavioral therapies to provide a "whole person" approach to treatment of substance-use disorders. Medications used in MAT are approved by the Federal Food and Drug Administration (FDA) and MAT programs are clinically driven and tailored to meet an individual patient's needs. MAT is primarily used for the treatment of opioid addiction such as heroin and prescription pain relievers that contain opioids. MAT is also used in alcohol-use disorder, and emerging therapies are forming for the treatment of methamphetamine use disorder. The goal of MAT is to support recovery and includes the ability to live a self-directed life. MAT operates to normalize brain chemistry, block euphoric effects from the substance of abuse, help curb physiological cravings, and helps to normalize body functions without the negative and euphoric effects of the substance(s) used.[18]	Medication-assisted treatment

are focused on education and treatment regimens to advance care and efficiency, including:

- Studies on the development of institutionalized regimens promote SUD treatment on a smaller scale, with the hopes of creating a system with applications to a broader spectrum population.[35]
- Studies evaluating the efficacy of inclusive SUD training for medical students aimed to encourage students to become active learners and advocates for SUD patients by addressing education on substance-use disorders and stigma. These studies showed favorable outcomes in reducing stigma-related bias in individuals receiving the training, which suggests a larger scale approach in training other potential members of SUD treatment teams may also show beneficial outcomes in stigma reduction and improvement of overall SUD treatment success.[36]
- Studies examining the efficacy of behavioral health and primary-care providers' treatment regimens found that intensive outpatient programs using initiatives to promote primary-care to their patients with SUD proved to be effective in those patients accessing and establishing care with a PCP.[37] Results also found that overall health outcomes are improved in those patients who follow regularly with a PCP.[37]

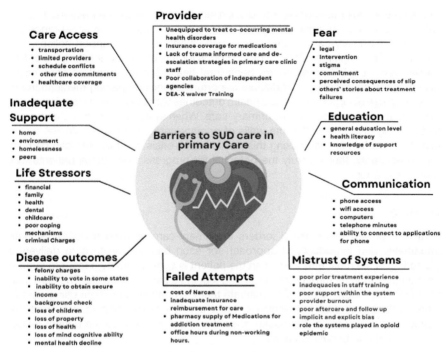

Provider
- Unequipped to treat co-occurring mental health disorders
- Insurance coverage for medications
- Lack of trauma informed care and de-escalation strategies in primary care clinic staff
- Poor collaboration of independent agencies
- DEA-X waiver Training

Care Access
- transportation
- limited providers
- schedule conflicts
- other time commitments
- healthcare coverage

Fear
- legal
- Intervention
- stigma
- commitment
- perceived consequences of slip
- others' stories about treatment failures

Inadequate Support
- home
- environment
- homelessness
- peers

Barriers to SUD care in primary Care

Education
- general education level
- health literacy
- knowledge of support resources

Life Stressors
- financial
- family
- health
- dental
- childcare
- poor coping mechanisms
- criminal Charges

Communication
- phone access
- wifi access
- computers
- telephone minutes
- ability to connect to applications for phone

Disease outcomes
- felony charges
- inability to vote in some states
- inability to obtain secure income
- background check
- loss of children
- loss of property
- loss of health
- loss of mind cognitive ability
- mental health decline

Failed Attempts
- cost of Narcan
- inadequate insurance reimbursement for care
- pharmacy supply of Medications for addiction treatment
- office hours during non-working hours.

Mistrust of Systems
- poor prior treatment experience
- inadequacies in staff training
- poor support within the system
- provider burnout
- poor aftercare and follow up
- implicit and explicit bias
- role the systems played in opioid epidemic

Fig. 1. Barriers to substance-use disorder care in primary-care.

By examining what treatment protocols can be replicated in primary-care, increased educational efforts of future physicians to reduce stigma, and the understanding that patients suffering from SUD generally have or develop multiple health conditions, role of the primary-care provider is even more crucial to the overall well-being of these patients, thus making the PCP an essential member of the interdisciplinary team in treating SUD.

Though SUD has been a continuously evolving topic for the past several decades, a great deal of stigma still exists. These often negative societal views and associated stigma of drug use limit patient interaction with behavioral health and health care providers, thus placing these marginalized patients in greater danger and further inhibits their prospect of a full and healthy life. Lastly, MAT providers also are often stigmatized by fellow health care colleagues. Physicians treating SUD are often scrutinized by physicians in other specialties due to the false view of MAT not serving as "real" medicine. Though these opinions are likely secondary to the regional stigma of SUD in general, these judgments may operate as a deterrent to providers to engage in further training and inhibit doctors from taking the steps to obtain their license to practice MAT, further widening the gap between patient and treatment. Programs aimed at deconstructing the stigma surrounding this topic are essential to overcoming the proliferative nature of SUD; for a complete list of barriers see **Fig. 1**.

DISCUSSION

Although the current landscape for the treatment of SUDs continues to perpetuate the very health disparities we strive to treat in primary-care, there are opportunities to consider. These roads potentially lead us to a more holistic and human-centered approach that includes a whole interdisciplinary team rather than a fractioned, "medicalized" approach. Treating substance-use disorders requires the acceptance and expansion of primary-care models that provide a framework to support holistic, integrated care and implementation of billing codes for this progress including the collaborative care model,[38] primary-care behavioral health model,[39] and comprehensive case management model.[40] Additional opportunities include pairing medications for substance-use disorder and related health outcomes with evidence-based, behavioral health treatment protocols within primary-care. When systems recognize that treating co-occurring disorders within the walls of primary-care can (and should be) a safe, sustainable option for addressing this public health crisis and this care can be reimbursed equitably, there is truly the potential for progress when these patients walk through the door.

SUMMARY

Treatment of substance-use disorders in primary-care requires a compassionate, empathetic, and individualized approach for each patient. Health care delivery in this setting is the most effective when the patient is surrounded by a team to support them on their journey through recovery and leading a self-directed life. The care team must identify personal biases and mitigate them, empower the patient using person-centered language and interventions, build a relationship upon mutual trust and respect, and be aware of the health disparities that exist to help the patient restore their physical and behavioral health.

This article presents the health care disparities that continue to perpetuate the stigma for treating patients with substance-use disorders in primary-care. It also serves to review the history of treating substance-use disorders in primary-care while looking at common medications used to treat SUDs and the laws and regulations that make these interventions possible. Although barriers remain for patients and providers, we have made progress in primary-care settings, including continuing to build a primary-care base that responds to the needs of the communities they serve. This includes recognizing that, for many regions of the United States, the health needs of the community are intricately related to the diagnosis and treatment of all-too-prevalent SUDs and their related behavioral and physical health problems. In this article, we hope to have described the pressing need to build strong interdisciplinary teams within primary-care and community partnerships (with addiction and mental health treatment facilities) to treat these vulnerable patients. By expanding access to care, working to reduce stigma (both of patients with SUD and stigma against their *peers* who treat SUD) while encouraging primary-care providers to train in and embrace the skills needed to effectively treat SUD, we see a future where the primary-care setting can be a place for healing and restoration of health that is not only possible, but is achievable for those suffering from SUDS.

CLINICS CARE POINTS

- Primary-care offices should train all staff and clinicians in mental health first aid and trauma-informed practices.
- Train providers on the utilization of the American Society of Addiction Medicine (ASAM) Level of Care Assessment to make treatment decisions.

- Primary-care practices should seek to build strong collaborations with addiction treatment and mental health centers so smooth transitions of care can be facilitated when a higher level is needed to be provided alongside primary-care.
- Partnerships with psychiatric services should be made available for all primary-care practices recognizing that co-occurring care is the norm, not the exception.
- All primary-care providers and behavioral health providers should be trained to treat co-occurring disorders and be ready to be co-occurring capable to align with the fourth edition of the ASAM Criteria release.
- Primary-care leadership systems should be educated about billing codes and care models that will reimburse equitably for interdisciplinary teams within primary-care while including behavioral health providers and people with lived experience as valuable members of the team.

To all the people in training, the future rests in your hands. This fight for a more equitable substance-use disorder treatment landscape is one we will have to demand from systems and payers, but the fight is worth it because we do it for those we love.

DISCLOSURE

Dr A.L. Colistra serves as a faculty member and consultant for the American Society of Addiction Medicine (ASAM) and is active in the development of the 4th edition of the ASAM criteria. A. Ward and E. Smith have no disclosures.

REFERENCES

1. NIDA. ADAPT-2 Trial Results Deliver a Breakthrough in Long Search for Methamphetamine Use Disorder Medication. National Institute on Drug Abuse website. 2021. Available at: https://nida.nih.gov/about-nida/noras-blog/2021/01/adapt-2-trial-results-deliver-breakthrough-in-long-search-methamphetamine-use-disorder-medication. Accessed October 30, 2022.
2. Office-Based Opioid-use Disorder (OUD) Treatment Billing | CMS. Available at: www.cms.gov   https://www.cms.gov/medicare/physician-fee-schedule/office-based-opioid-use-disorder-oud-treatment-billing. Accessed October 30, 2022.
3. American Psychiatric Association. Diagnostic and statistical manual of mental disorders. 1st ed. Washington, DC: American Psychiatric Association; 1952.
4. Norko MA, Fitch WL. DSM-5 and substance-use disorders: Clinicolegal implications. J Am Acad Psychiatry Law 2014. Available at: https://jaapl.org/content/42/4/443. Accessed October 20, 2022.
5. Robinson SM, Adinoff B. The classification of substance-use disorders: historical, contextual, and conceptual considerations. Behav Sci (Basel) 2016;6(3). https://doi.org/10.3390/bs6030018.
6. About the ASAM Criteria. Default. 2022. https://www.asam.org/asam-criteria/about-the-asam-criteria. [Accessed 20 October 2022].
7. Weisner C, Mertens J, Parthasarathy S, et al. Integrating primary medical care with addiction treatment: a randomized controlled trial. JAMA 2001;286(14): 1715–23.
8. Dorr H, Townley C. Integrating Substance-use Disorder Treatment and Primary-care – The National Academy for State Health Policy. https://www.nashp.org/integrating-substance-use-disorder-treatment-and-primary-care/. [Accessed 30 October 2022].

9. Saitz R, Larson MJ, Labelle C, et al. The case for chronic disease management for addiction. J Addict Med 2008;2(2):55–65.

10. Saitz R, Daaleman TP. Now is the time to address substance-use disorders in primary-care. Ann Fam Med 2017;15(4):306–8.

11. Barry CL, Huskamp HA. Moving beyond parity–mental health and addiction care under the ACA. N Engl J Med 2011;365(11):973–5.

12. Weaver MF, Jarvis MAE, Schnoll SH. Role of the Primary-care Physician in Problems of Substance Abuse. Arch Intern Med 1999;159(9):913–24.

13. Smith D. Virtual Mentor HISTORY OF MEDICINE The Evolution of Addiction Medicine as a Medical Specialty. Am Med Assoc J Ethics 2011;(13):900–5. Available at: https://journalofethics.ama-assn.org/sites/journalofethics.ama-assn.org/files/2018-05/mhst1-1112.pdf. Accessed October 30, 2022.

14. The ASAM Criteria. Available at: www.asam.org https://www.asam.org/asam-criteria.

15. Wesson DR, Smith DE. Buprenorphine in the treatment of opiate dependence. J Psychoactive Drugs 2010;42(2):161–75.

16. Division N. HHS Expands Access to Treatment for Opioid-use Disorder. HHS.gov. 2021. https://www.hhs.gov/about/news/2021/01/14/hhs-expands-access-to-treatment-for-opioid-use-disorder.html. [Accessed 20 October 2022].

17. Recovery Research Institute. Addictionary - Glossary of Substance-use Disorder Terminology. Recovery Research Institute. 2017. https://www.recoveryanswers.org/addiction-ary/. [Accessed 20 October 2022].

18. Chanell Baylor. Medication-Assisted treatment (MAT) | SAMHSA - Substance Abuse and Mental Health Services Administration. Samhsa.gov. 2021. https://www.samhsa.gov/medication-assisted-treatment. [Accessed 30 October 2022].

19. CDC. Health Disparities. Centers for Disease Control and Prevention. 2019. https://www.cdc.gov/aging/disparities/index.htm. [Accessed 20 October 2022].

20. What is the Definition of Addiction?. Available at: https://www.asam.org/quality-care/definition-of-addiction. Accessed October 24, 2022.

21. Primary-care | AAFP. Available at: https://www.aafp.org/about/policies/all/primary-care.html. Accessed October 24, 2022.

22. Primary health care. Available at: https://www.who.int/news-room/fact-sheets/detail/primary-health-care. Accessed October 24, 2022.

23. Peek CJ. Integrated behavioral health and primary-care: A common language. In: Talen MR, Burke Valeras A, editors. Integrated behavioral health in primary-care. 2013. p. 9–31. https://doi.org/10.1007/978-1-4614-6889-9_2. Springer New York.

24. Defining the PCMH | Agency for Health care Research and Quality. Available at: https://www.ahrq.gov/ncepcr/research/care-coordination/pcmh/define.html. Accessed October 24, 2022.

25. Team-Based Care Toolkit | Patient and Interprofessional Education | ACP. Available at: https://www.acponline.org/practice-resources/patient-and-interprofessional-education/team-based-care-toolkit. Accessed October 24, 2022.

26. Social Determinants of Health - Healthy People 2030 | health.gov. Available at: https://health.gov/healthypeople/priority-areas/social-determinants-health. Accessed October 24, 2022.

27. Substance Abuse and Mental Health Services Administration. SAMHSA's concept of trauma and guidance for a trauma-informed approach. HHS Publication No. (SMA). Rockville, MD: Substance Abuse and Mental Health Services Administration; 2014. p. 14–4884.

28. APA Dictionary of Psychology. Available at: https://dictionary.apa.org/stigma. Accessed October 24, 2022.

29. Vela MB, Erondu AI, Smith NA, et al. Eliminating explicit and implicit biases in health care: evidence and research needs. Annu Rev Public Health 2022;43: 477–501.

30. Centers of excellence. Department of Human Services. Available at: https://www. dhs.pa.gov/Services/Assistance/Pages/Centers-of-Excellence.aspx.   Accessed October 24, 2022.

31. Lyon J. SAMHSA Releases New State-By-State Reports on US Behavioral Health. JAMA 2017;318(12):1098.

32. About Us. Available at: https://www.asam.org/about-us. Accessed October 24, 2022.

33. Substance Abuse and Mental Health Services Administration. Key substance-use and mental health indicators in the United States: Results from the 2020 National Survey on Drug Use and Health (HHS Publication No. PEP21-07-01-003, NSDUH Series H-56). Rockville (MD): Center for Behavioral Health Statistics and Quality, Substance Abuse and Mental Health Services Administration; 2021. Available at: https://www.samhsa.gov/data/.

34. McCuistian C, Burlew K, Espinosa A, et al. Advancing health equity through substance-use research. J Psychoactive Drugs 2021;1–5. https://doi.org/10. 1080/02791072.2021.1994673.

35. Codell N, Kelley AT, Jones AL, et al. Aims, development, and early results of an interdisciplinary primary-care initiative to address patient vulnerabilities. Am J Drug Alcohol Abuse 2021;47(2):160–9.

36. Cantone RE, Hanneman NS, Chan MG, et al. Effects of implementing an interactive substance-use disorders workshop on a family medicine clerkship. Fam Med 2021;53(4):295–9.

37. Wasserman R, Terrien J. Integration of primary-care into the substance-use disorder outpatient treatment setting. J Am Assoc Nurse Pract 2020;33(8):652–60.

38. Collaborative Care | University of Washington AIMS Center. aims.uw.edu. Available at: http://aims.uw.edu/collaborative-care. Accessed October 30, 2022.

39. Reiter JT, Dobmeyer AC, Hunter CL. The primary-care behavioral health (PCBH) model: an overview and operational definition. J Clin Psychol Med Settings 2018; 25(2):109–26.

40. TIP 27: Comprehensive case management for substance abuse treatment | SAMHSA publications. Samhsa.gov. 2015. https://store.samhsa.gov/product/ TIP-27-Comprehensive-Case-Management-for-Substance-Abuse-Treatment/ SMA15-4215. [Accessed 20 October 2022].

ACE

"What Happened to You" Screening for Adverse Childhood Experiences or Trauma-Informed Care

Courtney Barry, PsyD, MS[a,*], Constance Gundacker, MD, MPH[b]

KEYWORDS

- Trauma-informed care • ACEs • Trauma • Trauma-informed approaches
- Primary care

KEY POINTS

- Exposure to potentially traumatic events is common and can have lasting adverse influences on a person's well-being.
- Trauma is prevalent, even in primary care practice, with rates ranging from 57% to 87.8%.
- Trauma-informed care can use different trauma-specific strategies, such as screening or universal trauma precautions, which allow providers to use different approaches (communication strategies) without knowing a person's trauma history.
- Screening using a trauma-informed approach can lead to a deeper understanding of factors affecting patients' health and allow for early detection, more impactful and targeted assessments and plans, and intervention as needed.

INTRODUCTION

Each day many people experience potentially traumatic events. This can range from witnessing someone getting hurt, being in a motor vehicle accident, or even being put down by another person. Some events may affect an individual for a short period, for instance, until the traumatic event is over, whereas others may have a lasting impact on individuals. To understand and address potentially traumatic events, we must have a foundational definition of what is trauma. According to the Substance Abuse Mental Health Services Administration, "Trauma results from an event, series of events, or set of circumstances that is experienced by an individual as physically or emotionally harmful or threatening and that has lasting adverse effects on the individual's functioning and physical, social, emotional, or spiritual well-being."[1] Primary

[a] Department of Psychiatry and Behavioral Medicine, Medical College of Wisconsin, 8701 West Watertown Plank Road, Milwaukee, WI 53226, USA; [b] Department of Pediatrics, Medical College of Wisconsin, Children's Corporate Center, Suite C730, 999 North 92nd Street, Milwaukee, WI 53226, USA
* Corresponding author.
E-mail address: cobarry@mcw.edu

Prim Care Clin Office Pract 50 (2023) 71–82
https://doi.org/10.1016/j.pop.2022.10.003
0095-4543/23/© 2022 Elsevier Inc. All rights reserved.

care providers play an essential role in reducing the impact of potentially traumatic and traumatic experiences through early identification, education, referrals as needed, and the provision of trauma-informed care (TIC) to prevent retraumatization.

Types of Trauma

Throughout an individual's life, a person can experience different types of events that are traumatic. **Table 1** highlights different traumas that can occur in childhood and adulthood:

Trauma influences on health through the life span

Social and physical environments affect health and development across generations.[3] These environments are especially important during critical/sensitive periods of development. Neural plasticity or the brain's ability to change or reorganize based on stimuli is highest in the first 3 years of life and then again during adolescence.[3,4] Positive or negative experiences during the first 3 years of life are critical to early brain development and lay the foundation for future physical, developmental, and social/emotional health.

Individual response to the same life experience varies due to not only genetic variability but also based on differential exposure to social and environmental protective and risk factors. The most important protective factor and mitigator of negative childhood life experiences is a safe, stable, nurturing relationship (SSNR) because it buffers children's stress response to negative life experiences. For most children, a parent or caregiver is the source of this SSNR (may also be a coach, teacher).[5,6] Negative life experiences can result in 3 different types of stress responses: positive, tolerable, or toxic. These different types of stress responses result in differing levels of activation of the hypothalamic-pituitary-adrenocortical axis and the sympathetic-adrenomedullary systems, resulting in differing levels of stress hormones such as cortisol, norepinephrine, and adrenaline.[3,4]

- *Positive stress responses* result from a brief and mild/moderate stressful event with a short activation of the stress response system and a quick return to normal with the support of a SSNR.
  ○ Examples of positive stress responses include stress associated with taking a test or receiving a childhood immunization.
- *Tolerable stress responses* are associated with exposure to more severe nonnormative experiences. These experiences result in greater activation of the stress response system but in the setting of a buffering SSNR, prolonged and/or excessive activation of the stress response system can be mitigated.
  ○ Examples include a natural disaster or the death of a family member.
- *Toxic stress responses* result from excessive and prolonged activation of the stress response system in the absence of buffering SSNRs. Excessive and prolonged activation of the stress response system leads to physiologic dysregulations that affect health and development across the life span.
  ○ Examples include physical or sexual abuse, or neglect.

Resilience can also help mitigate negative outcomes of adverse childhood experiences (ACEs). Resilience is the ability to adapt positively despite significant adversities.[5,7] Resilience is a dynamic process and is supported through adaptational mechanisms of human development, which can be remembered through the mnemonic THREADS (Thinking and learning brain and opportunity for cognitive development), hope for future self, regulation (self-regulation and self-control), efficacy (self-efficacy), attachment (Secure attachment with SSNR), development (achieving age-appropriate developmental tasks), social (supportive network of healthy relationships).[5]

Table 1
Examples of types of trauma

Childhood Trauma		Adult Trauma	
Physical abuse	Family member attempt or commit suicide	Domestic violence	Emotional/ psychological abuse
Sexual abuse	Violence in the community	Sexual abuse	Unexpected loss of a family member
Emotional/ psychological abuse	Incarcerated family members	Physical abuse	Torture
Substance abuse in family members	Bullying	Serious medical events	Combat trauma
Parents who have mental health conditions	Medical trauma	Natural disasters	Community violence
Parental separation	Trafficking	Terrorism/mass violence	Witnessing someone getting hurt or killed
This is not an exhaustive list of the different types of traumas that can occur within childhood and adulthood			

Data from Refs.[1,2]

Potentially traumatic events that occur in childhood (0–17 years) are called ACEs. A foundational study completed by the Center for Disease Control and Kaiser Permanente examined different categories of ACEs.[8] Results indicated 52% of adults experienced more than 1 category of ACEs, whereas 6.2% reported 4 or more different categories of experiences.[8] An important finding of this study was a graded-dose–response relationship related between ACEs and health. Individuals who reported 4 or more ACEs had almost 4 times higher risk of health conditions, such as chronic bronchitis and were almost twice as likely to develop diabetes.[8] This important study demonstrates how trauma, even in childhood, can affect an individual in adulthood.

Traumatic events can occur in adulthood as well. Individuals who experience trauma in childhood may be more likely to experience trauma in adulthood.[9] This may be due to individuals who have been a victim of a previous trauma, have a higher rate of experiencing revictimization.[10] Research now has shown that trauma occurring in adulthood between the ages of 18 and 61 years is having an effect on an individual's health later in life.[11] This demonstrates the importance of considering how trauma even in adulthood can continue to affect a person's health and well-being.

Trauma Prevalence

Trauma is common globally and within the United States. The prevalence of individuals experiencing at least one traumatic event is 70.4% globally, 60% to 90% within the United States, which is the same rate within a primary care setting, and 50% to 70% for children aged younger than 18 years.[9,12–17] About 27.9% of individuals globally and 53% of primary care patients have experienced 4 or more traumas.[12,14] With the high prevalence of trauma, it is important for primary care providers (PCPs) to be cognizant of trauma within their patient population.

Trauma-Informed Care

To treat patients who have experienced a trauma, it is important to take a trauma-informed approach to care. TIC is an approach to care that[18]:

- "Realizes the widespread impact of trauma and understands potential paths for recovery;
- Recognizes the signs and symptoms of trauma in clients, families, staff, and others involved with the system;
- Responds by fully integrating knowledge about trauma into policies, procedures, and practices;
- Seeks to actively resist retraumatization."

TIC uses 6 guiding principles (**Table 2**), which are generalizable and help to inform different trauma-informed practices and approaches.

TIC is an approach that moves from "What is wrong with you" to "What happened to you?" to "What is strong with you?"[5,19] It encourages organizations to understand an individual's past and present in order to provide support and healing. In health care, this may look like realizing that a patient may have an underlying trauma history, which prevents them from attending their appointments. By using a TIC approach to care, it can improve patient outcomes with their treatment and also reduce provider burnout.[20]

Trauma-informed care in health care

There are different TIC domains that can be used in health care settings, including universal trauma precautions and trauma-specific strategies as seen in **Table 3**.[20]

The American Academy of Family Physicians (AAFP) and the American Academy of Pediatrics (AAP) recognize the importance of TIC and have recommended that all family physicians and pediatric medical providers use a trauma-informed approach in all patient encounters, regardless of whether or not they have disclosed a trauma history.[21,22] Using a public health approach, this includes 3 tiers[22]:

1. Primary prevention: assess and address social determinants of health, relational health, and resilience factor promotion.
2. Secondary prevention: promote protective factors and child/family resilience, parent/caregiver awareness of trauma, involve families in program development and evaluation.
3. Tertiary prevention: trauma-informed therapies for symptomatic children/youth.

The AAFP also identified 4 strategies in working with adults who have a history of childhood trauma[21]:

1. Warn patients before asking invasive or potentially upsetting questions.
2. Ask permission before initiating touch or physical examination and explain what you are doing.
3. Use caring, sensitive language, such as "Some people find it helpful to take a few deep, relaxing breaths" versus "You need to relax."
4. Assure patients that any information they share will be kept confidential.

Screening in Primary Care

Screening for trauma can help providers understand a patient's history, and ultimately how to provide care that prevents retraumatization and promotes healing. Through screening, providers can begin to have a conversation about their score and what it means, regarding the patient's care. Despite the prevalence of trauma, screening uptake in the primary care setting has been relatively slow. A study assessed the

Table 2 Guiding principles	
Principle	**Description**
Safety	Employees within an organization and those that they serve feel physically and psychologically safe
Trustworthiness and transparency	The organization is transparent in their decision and works to build trust not only with individuals they serve but also with staff
Peer support	Individuals who are trauma survivors are a part of the organization and important in providing services
Collaboration and mutuality	Shared decision-making occurs not only between staff but individuals the organization serves
Empowerment and choice	Recognizing strengths of staff and the individuals the organization serves and allowing the individuals to have choices in their treatment plan, in order to heal
Cultural, historical, and gender issues	Acknowledging, addressing, and moving forward from stereotypes, biases, and historical trauma, which includes having policies and practices that are open to the different cultural, gender, and ethnic needs of the individuals the organization serves

Data from Substance Abuse and Mental Health Services Administration. SAMHSA's Concept of Trauma and Guidance for a Trauma-Informed Approach. HHS Publication No. (SMA) 14-4884. Rockville, MD: Substance Abuse and Mental Health Services Administration, 2014.

screening practices of family physicians and found that 29.6% of providers always or usually screen patients for trauma in childhood.[23] As part of their role, 79% of the physicians thought screening for childhood trauma was a part of their responsibilities, although they thought that the biggest barriers to screening for childhood trauma were time to provide support or inquire about a trauma history.[23] To overcome these barriers, a study found that screening before the visit indicated a trauma prevalence within the patient population and PCPs were more likely to talk to patients about their trauma history if they had more than 1 ACE.[24]

In the 2013 AAP Periodic Survey, only 4% of pediatricians usually asked about all 7 ACEs from the original ACE study and 32% did not usually ask about any. The mostly commonly asked about ACEs by pediatricians were maternal depression (46%) and parental separation/divorce (42%).[25] Reported barriers to providers screening include lack of knowledge about ACE study and trauma, knowledge or availability of resources for positive screen, and lack of time.[5,25,26] However, 2 feasibility studies within primary care revealed time was not a significant barrier.[24,27] Lack of knowledge can be addressed through education as part of a quality improvement project implementing ACE screening within a primary care setting.[28]

Adult patient
Screening adult patients for trauma can help providers understand how their past trauma history may affect their child's health. For example, if a patient is using substances to cope with their trauma history, providers can use this information to address behavioral change and educate on how the substance use may be affecting their child's health. It may also give providers an opportunity to educate the patient on why they engage or do not engage in certain behaviors, which may be connected to

Table 3
Trauma-informed care

Principle	Description	In a Clinical Setting
Universal Trauma Precautions		
Patient-centered communication and care	Using small changes in clinical practice to build trust with patients, without knowing if a patient does or does not have a trauma history	• Telling a patient you will be putting your hand on them, in order to complete the physical examination • Allowing a patient to use a hand signal or a word if they are feeling uncomfortable at any point during an examination • Ask the patient if there are certain concerns they would like to address during the appointment • Encourage questions and ask about any worries or concerns and how you can help (eg, leaving door ajar)
Understanding the health effects of trauma	Providers have an understanding that unhealthy coping skills may be the result of a trauma history	• Use empathetic listening when patients discuss maladaptive coping behaviors, such as alcohol or smoking • Understand that an unhealthy coping skill may be prohibiting the patient from following up with appointments, instead of labeling the patient as noncompliant
Trauma-Specific Strategies		
Interprofessional collaboration	Collaborating with other professionals to provide resources and referrals for patients who disclose or have a trauma history	• Identify other providers who have experience in working with patients with a trauma history • Conduct a warm hand-off with other providers for a patient with a trauma history
Understanding your own history and reactions	Providers should be aware of their own trauma history and their reactions (and how they cope) when hearing about trauma stories from their patients	• Identify signs and symptoms of burnout • Engage in self-care when working with patients who have a trauma history

(continued on next page)

Table 3 (continued)		
Principle	**Description**	**In a Clinical Setting**
Screening	Assessing patients for a trauma history, either current or in past, to understand a patient's trauma history	• Provide an introductory statement to screening • Determine if screening will be in-person or use self-report measures • Identify resources if a patient has a positive screen • Provide education to all staff when discussing results of the screen

Adapted from Raja S, Hasnain M, Hoersch M, Gove-Yin S, Rajagopalan C. Trauma informed care in medicine: current knowledge and future research directions. Fam Community Health. 2015;38(3):216-226.

their trauma history. This may help patients build trust in their providers.[29] Screening for trauma may also allow providers to initiate referrals to begin to address their underlying trauma and ultimately provide integrative care to the patient (addressing the physical and mental health). The difficulty in screening is that patients may experience recall bias, where they may not recall a traumatic event during their life. Furthermore, providers may be hesitant fearing that patients will experience discomfort with answering the questions; however, research indicates that patients did not find screening for ACEs invasive.[29]

Screening for adults during a clinical encounter can be important; however, there are different areas to consider before screening patients:

- *Time:* When screening, providers need to consider the length of interaction time with patients and if they will be assessing current trauma or past trauma.[20]
  - Screening a patient for trauma has not shown to lengthen the clinical visit.[21]
- *Positive screen:* Providers should also consider what they will do with the results of the screening, such as how they may change their practice to be more trauma-informed or what referrals or support they will provide to the patient.[21]
  - Using community connections so that patients have access to various services they may need.[21]
  - To implement a screening tool, it is important to educate all clinic staff on working with a patient who does screen positive.[20]
  - Consider using trauma-informed language both in documentation and in patient encounters.[21]
- *Screening tool:* The provider should choose a screening tool that fits their practice and provides information that can be used to provide TIC.
  - Training of all staff and providers needs to occur before initiation of screening in order to ensure screening is done in a trauma-informed approach and appropriate referrals are made when necessary.
  - Providing education on ACEs and trauma and how different aspects of a clinical encounter may change.[21]

Pediatric patient

The AAP advocates pediatric health care providers to screen for potentially traumatic events, ACEs, and resilience during well-childcare visits. This may take a variety of approaches depending on the medical practice and includes both surveillance and screening. Surveillance that is less formal than screening should happen at every patient encounter. Surveillance may include identification of protective and risk factors during the history, potential trauma symptoms during the review of systems, and potential trauma signs on physical examination. Trauma should also always be considered in the differential diagnosis. If child safety concerns develop, mandatory reporting is required to child protective services.[5]

When considering screening for potentially traumatic experiences and ACEs within pediatric primary care, it is important to take a family-centered approach. SSNRs are the most important buffer for toxic stress; therefore, providing education and support for the primary caregiver in addition to the child is essential.[6] There are a variety of things to consider when approaching formal screening during the pediatric patient encounter[5, 26]:

- *Target population to screen:* When a primary care provider is seeing a pediatric patient for a clinical visit, formal screening can occur with the patient (age-appropriate and dependent) and/or with the primary caregiver.
  - ○ *Pediatric patient target of screener:* Formal screening of the pediatric patient can include trauma-specific screeners if trauma experience is known, resilience screening, and/or consideration of trauma as a differential diagnosis for nontrauma-specific screening tools used in pediatric primary care.
  - ○ *Primary caregiver target of screener:* Screening parents/caregivers for ACEs during pediatric medical visits offers the opportunity for a deeper conversation on issues that might be affecting parenting styles, which has a direct influence on the attachment relationship and the ability of a child to develop resilience in the face of adversity. Parental ACEs have been linked to concerning outcomes in children. Some clinics have found implementing parental ACE screening and asking for aggregate ACEs (rather than identifying specific ACEs) results in more accurate and higher reporting of parental ACEs. This has the potential to allow for a discussion on issues that impact parenting and provide parenting resources and other community supports as needed.[5, 26]
- *Types of Screeners:* Many pediatric primary care clinics already have screening tools implemented for development, mental health, or social needs (eg, PHQ-9, ASQ, Edinburgh, PSC, social determinants of health screeners). Results of these commonly used screeners can be used to identify strengths and risk factors (eg, social determinants of health screeners, Edinburgh) or symptoms or sequela of potential trauma (eg, PHQ-9, ASQ). Trauma-specific screeners also exist for pediatric patients if trauma exposure is known or expected. There are also a few standardized validated resilience screening tools that can be considered.[5]
- *Family-centered discussion:* No matter the approach, the goal of screening is to open a discussion with the family. Screening identifies potential risk and protective factors and can help a conversation with the family on potential strengths to build on and early intervention as needed to appropriate resources.[26]
- *Response to positive surveillance or screen:* The response by pediatric providers to a positive surveillance or screen for a potentially traumatic event depends on the level of exposure (single vs cumulative, minor vs major) and the amount of trauma symptoms (none, mild, moderate, or severe). The pediatric provider's response might include trauma-informed anticipatory guidance and education, close monitoring, and/or referrals to community services or mental health as needed.[5] Primary care providers should not underestimate the power of compassionate listening and understanding because trauma survivors think

Table 4
Screeners for trauma and Post-Traumatic Stress Disorder (PTSD)

Name of Screener	Number of Items	Target Population?	Person Completing the Screener
Trauma Symptom Checklist for Children[30]	54 items	Children (8–16 years)	Completed by parent/caregiver
Center for Youth Wellness ACE Questionnaire for Children and Adolescents[31]	17 items: Children 19 items: Adolescents	Children (0–12 years; 13–19 years)	Completed by parent/caregiver Adolescents: Self-report or completed by parent/caregiver
Child and Adolescent Trauma Screen[32]	40 items	Children (3–6 years); 7–17 years	Self-report (aged 7–17 years)/completed by caregiver (3–17 years)
Primary Care PTSD Screen for DSM-5*[33]	5 items	Adults	Self-report
Pediatric ACEs and Related Life-events Screener[34]	17 items for child 19 items for adolescent self-report	Children (0–11 years)/adolescents (12–19 years)	Self-report/completed by parent
Child PTSD Symptom Scale for DSM-5[35]	27 items: Interview	Children/adolescents (8–18 years)	Clinician/therapist Self-report
Child Trauma Screen[36]	10 items	Children/adolescents (6–17 years)	Clinician/staff
PTSD Checklist for DSM-5*[37]	20 items	Adults	Self-report
Structured Trauma-Related Experiences and Symptoms Screener[38]	83 items	Adults	Self-report
UCLA PTSD Reaction Index Brief Form[39]	11 items	Children and Youth 7–17 years in the study	Self-report

*Diagnostic and Statistical Manual of Mental Disorders Fifth Edition (DSM-5)

this is one of the most important factors for healing.[26] Additionally, in one study parents were asked about needed or desired resources. The most common needed resource was parenting resources and support and information was the second, both of which the primary care pediatric provider is qualified to provide.[27]

It is important for providers to be familiar with the screeners available and what may be best for their patients and practice (**Table 4**).

SUMMARY

Early recognition of potentially traumatic events during childhood can lead to appropriate anticipatory guidance and referrals as needed to buffer the experience, prevent toxic stress, and prevent negative long-term health outcomes. Helping adults understand the potential influence ACEs have had on their current health and parenting practices can lead to a more targeted approach to addressing current health needs and provision of parental resource supports to interrupt the cycle of intergenerational trauma. Primary care providers are essential players in addressing and preventing trauma.

CLINICS CARE POINTS

- Always consider trauma as part of the differential diagnosis.
- The goal of screening for trauma or ACEs is not to diagnose but rather to identify risk and serve as a starting point for a deeper patient-centered conversation.
- When choosing a screening tool, choose one that best fits your practice and need. Make sure that staff is trained on how to respond to a positive screen.
- Discussions on trauma and ACEs should always be paired with discussions on protective factors, strengths, and resilience. Ensure you have the appropriate resources to refer a patient for further treatment.
- When seeing patients that have been labeled as "noncompliant," "difficult," or with frequent "no-shows," reframe your thinking from "What is wrong with you" to "What happened to you?" to "What is strong with you?"

DISCLOSURE

The authors have no financial or commercial conflicts of interest to disclose.

REFERENCES

1. Substance Abuse and Mental Health Services Administration. Trauma-informed care in behavioral health services. Treatment improvement protocol (TIP) Series 57. HHS Publication No. (SMA) 13-4801. Rockville, MD: Substance Abuse and Mental Health Services Administration; 2014.
2. Center for Disease Control. Adverse childhood experiences. In: Adverse childhood experiences. 2022. Available at: https://www.cdc.gov/violenceprevention/aces/index.html. Accessed April 16, 2022.
3. Shonkoff JP, Garner AS, Committee on Psychosocial Aspects of C, et al. The lifelong effects of early childhood adversity and toxic stress. Pediatrics 2012;129(1):e232–46.

4. National Scientific Council on the Developing Child. Excessive stress disrupts the architecture of the developing brain: working paper 3. Updated Edition 2005/2014. Available at: http://www.developingchild.harvard.edu. Accessed April 29 2022.

5. Forkey H, Szilagyi M, Kelly ET, et al. Trauma-informed care. Pediatrics 2021; 148(2). https://doi.org/10.1542/peds.2021-052580 [published Online First: Epub Date]|.

6. Center for Disease Control and Prevention. Essentials for childhood: creating Safe, stable, nurturing relationships and environments. In Child abuse and neglect. Available at: https://www.cdc.gov/violenceprevention/childabuseandneglect/essentials.html. Accessed April 29, 2022.

7. Masten AS. Ordinary magic. Resilience processes in development. Am Psychol 2001;56(3):227–38.

8. Felitti VJ, Anda RF, Nordenberg D, et al. Relationship of childhood abuse and household dysfunction to many of the leading causes of death in adults. The Adverse Childhood Experiences (ACE) Study. Am J Prev Med 1998;14(4): 245–58.

9. Bürgin D, Boonmann C, Schmeck K, et al. Compounding stress: childhood adversity as a risk factor for adulthood trauma exposure in the health and retirement study. J Trauma Stress 2021;34(1):124–36.

10. Widom CS, Czaja SJ, Dutton MA. Childhood victimization and lifetime revictimization. Child Abuse Negl 2008;32(8):785–96.

11. Krause N, Shaw BA, Cairney J. A descriptive epidemiology of lifetime trauma and the physical health status of older adults. Psychol Aging 2004;19(4):637–48.

12. Kessler RC, Aguilar-Gaxiola S, Alonso J, et al. Trauma and PTSD in the WHO World Mental Health Surveys. Eur J Psychotraumatol 2017;8(sup5):1353383.

13. Alim TN, Graves E, Mellman TA, et al. Trauma exposure, posttraumatic stress disorder and depression in an African-American primary care population. J Natl Med Assoc 2006;98(10):1630–6.

14. Kalmakis KA, Shafer MB, Chandler GE, et al. Screening for childhood adversity among adult primary care patients. J Am Assoc Nurse Pract 2018;30(4):193–200.

15. Greene T, Neria Y, Gross R. Prevalence, detection and correlates of PTSD in the primary care setting: a systematic review. J Clin Psychol Med Settings 2016; 23(2):160–80.

16. Holman EA, Silver RC, Waitzkin H. Traumatic life events in primary care patients: a study in an ethnically diverse sample. Arch Fam Med 2000;9(9):802–10.

17. Gillespie CF, Bradley B, Mercer K, et al. Trauma exposure and stress-related disorders in inner city primary care patients. Gen Hosp Psychiatry 2009;31(6): 505–14.

18. Substance Abuse and Mental Health Services Administration. SAMHSA's Concept of trauma and guidance for a trauma-informed approach. HHS publication No. (SMA) 14-4884. Rockville, MD: Substance Abuse and Mental Health Services Administration; 2014.

19. Center for Health Care Strategies. What is Trauma-Informed Care?. In: What is Trauma-Informed Care?. 2021. Available at. https://www.traumainformedcare.chcs.org/what-is-trauma-informed-care/. Accessed April 16 2022.

20. Raja S, Hasnain M, Hoersch M, et al. Trauma informed care in medicine: current knowledge and future research directions. Fam Community Health 2015;38(3): 216–26.

21. Leasy M, O'Gurek DT, Savoy ML. Unlocking clues to current health in past history: childhood trauma and healing. Fam Pract Manag 2019;26(2):5–10.

22. Duffee J, Szilagyi M, Forkey H, et al. Trauma-Informed Care in Child Health Systems. Pediatrics 2021;148(2). https://doi.org/10.1542/peds.2021-052579 [published Online First: Epub Date]|.

23. Weinreb L, Savageau JA, Candib LM, et al. Screening for childhood trauma in adult primary care patients: a cross-sectional survey. Prim Care Companion CNS Disord 2010;12(6):26831.

24. Glowa PT, Olson AL, Johnson DJ. Screening for adverse childhood experiences in a family medicine setting: a feasibility study. J Am Board Fam Med 2016;29(3): 303–7.

25. Kerker BD, Storfer-Isser A, Szilagyi M, et al. Do pediatricians ask about adverse childhood experiences in pediatric primary care? Acad Pediatr 2016;16(2): 154–60.

26. Gillespie RJ. Screening for adverse childhood experiences in pediatric primary care: pitfalls and possibilities. Pediatr Ann 2019;48(7):e257–61.

27. Gillespie RJ, Folger AT. Feasibility of assessing parental ACEs in pediatric primary care: implications for practice-based implementation. J Child Adolesc Trauma 2017;10(3):249–56.

28. Bryant C, VanGraafeiland B. Screening for adverse childhood experiences in primary care: a quality improvement project. J Pediatr Health Care 2020;34(2): 122–7.

29. Rariden C, SmithBattle L, Yoo JH, et al. Screening for adverse childhood experiences: literature review and practice implications. J Nurse Pract 2021;17(1): 98–104.

30. Nilsson D, Wadsby M, Svedin CG. The psychometric properties of the trauma symptom checklist for children (TSCC) in a sample of Swedish children. Child Abuse Negl 2008;32(6):627–36.

31. Burke Harris N, Renschler T. Center for youth wellness ACE-questionnaire (CYW ACE-Q child, teen, teen SR). San Francisco, CA: Center for Youth Wellness; 2015.

32. Sachser C, Berliner L, Holt T, et al. International development and psychometric properties of the Child and Adolescent Trauma Screen (CATS). J Affect Disord 2017;210:189–95.

33. Prins A, Bovin MJ, Smolenski DJ, et al. The Primary Care PTSD Screen for DSM-5 (PC-PTSD-5): Development and Evaluation Within a Veteran Primary Care Sample. J Gen Intern Med 2016;31(10):1206–11.

34. Thakur N, Hessler D, Koita K, et al. Pediatrics adverse childhood experiences and related life events screener (PEARLS) and health in a safety-net practice. Child Abuse Negl 2020;108:104685.

35. Foa EB, Asnaani A, Zang Y, et al. Psychometrics of the Child PTSD Symptom Scale for DSM-5 for Trauma-Exposed Children and Adolescents. J Clin Child Adolesc Psychol 2018;47(1):38–46.

36. Lang JM, Connell CM. Development and validation of a brief trauma screening measure for children: the child trauma screen. Psychol Trauma 2017;9(3):390–8.

37. Blevins CA, Weathers FW, Davis MT, et al. The posttraumatic stress disorder checklist for DSM-5 (PCL-5): development and initial psychometric evaluation. J Trauma Stress 2015;28(6):489–98.

38. Grasso DJ, Felton JW, Reid-Quinones K. The structured trauma-related experiences and symptoms screener (STRESS): development and preliminary psychometrics. Child Maltreat 2015;20(3):214–20.

39. Rolon-Arroyo B, Oosterhoff B, Layne CM, et al. The UCLA PTSD reaction index for DSM-5 brief form: a screening tool for trauma-exposed youths. J Am Acad Child Adolesc Psychiatry 2020;59(3):434–43.

Adjustment Disorder
Diagnosis and Treatment in Primary Care

Kamini Geer, MD, MPH

KEYWORDS

• Adjustment disorder • Background • Stressors • Reaction • Diagnosis • Treatment

KEY POINTS

• The diagnosis of adjustment disorder is defined by either the Diagnostic and Statistical Manual V or the ICD-11.
• There are factors that put individuals more at risk for adjustment disorder.
• There are psychological and pharmacologic therapies available for adjustment disorder.

CASE

EP has been a patient in your family medicine clinic for many years. She is a 57-year-old woman with a history of well-controlled diabetes mellitus type 2 and hypertension. During the pandemic, her employment shifted her to working from home, and she had been doing very well with this. Today she comes in with a complaint of 1 month of intermittent uncontrollable episodes of excessive worrying, shaking, and crying fits. She also reports difficulty falling asleep at night. All these episodes are associated with either interactions with or thoughts of her downstairs neighbor. EP has lived for several years on the top floor of a three story apartment buidling. She has always enjoyed a good relationship with all the neighbors in her building. Three months ago, a new downstairs neighbor moved in and has begun to complain about the noise level from EP's apartment. This neighbor has submitted several noise complaints against EP with building management, and EP has been given a warning that if the noise level does not improve, she will be evicted. The neighbor will also bang on the floor of her apartment at random times during the day. EP does not believe she is being too noisy, and the complaints, threat of eviction, and random banging on her floors has "put her on edge." Her episodes coincide with interactions with this neighbor, and even with walking by this neighbor's door. These new symptoms have also started to influence her performance at work and her interactions with her family. She even feels like she cannot relax in her home. She has come to you, her primary care physician, to ask for assistance with these symptoms. *What does she have? What can you do to assist?*

AdventHealth East Orlando Family Medicine Residency, 7975 Lake Underhill Road Suite 210, Orlando, FL 32822, USA
E-mail address: kamini.geer.md@adventhealth.com

Prim Care Clin Office Pract 50 (2023) 83–88
https://doi.org/10.1016/j.pop.2022.10.006
0095-4543/23/© 2022 Elsevier Inc. All rights reserved.

primarycare.theclinics.com

Background

Adjustment Disorder first appeared in the Diagnostic and Statistical Manual (DSM) I in 1952 as "Transient Situational Personality Disorder." During the next few years, it was given different names until 1980, when the term "Adjustment Disorder" was introduced in the DSM III.[1] There have been varying changes to the definition and categorization of the diagnosis over the iterations of the DSM,[2] until the most recent definition in the DSM 5.[1,2] In addition to being defined in the DSM V, adjustment disorder is also defined in the ICD-11.[1,2] There are similarities and differences between these diagnostic criteria.

Definition

There are 5 basic diagnostic criterion for adjustment disorder in the DSM V: emotion or behavioral symptoms within 3 months of identifiable stressor(s), symptoms are clinically significant and out of proportion to normal reactions to stressor according to social or cultural context, symptoms do not represent normal bereavement, stress-related disturbance does not meet the criteria for another mental disorder and is not merely an exacerbation of a preexisting mental disorder and once the stressor (or its consequences) has terminated, the symptoms do not persist for more than an additional 6 months.[1,2]

The DSM V also divides adjustment disorder into 6 different subtypes depending on what is the presenting symptom. The types are outlined in **Table 1**.[1]

There has been criticism of these categorizations of adjustment disorder in that research has not clearly demonstrated a clear distinction of these symptoms in those with adjustment disorder because often these symptoms can coexist at the same time. As a result, adjustment disorder is more often seen as a unidimensional disorder that is more clearly defined by the ICD-11 diagnostic criteria.[3]

The ICD-11 Diagnostic Criteria are as Follows

- identifiable stressor(s)
- maladaptive reactions that occur within 1 month after exposure to stressor and tend to resolve within 6 months if the stressor has ended
- symptoms of preoccupation and failure to adapt related with the identified stressor and interfere with everyday functioning
- symptoms do not justify another mental or behavioral disorder

A comparison of these 2 diagnostic criteria demonstrate similarities in that there must be a stressor, there is a reaction to the stressor that affects the ability of the patient to function in her or his everyday life, the symptoms are not severe enough to warrant another psychiatric diagnosis, and the symptoms will resolve within 6 months or earlier if the stressor is removed.[3]

A meta-analysis conducted to determine those most at risk for adjustment disorder demonstrated that female gender, unemployed status, low income, low social support, and a history of mental health disorders predicted adjustment disorders compared with no mental health condition.[4] In addition, those with adjustment disorders tended to perceive events as more stressful than those without a mental health condition but this perception did not differ from those with depression or exhaustion disorder.[4] Individuals with a history of abuse or neglect were also more at risk for adjustment disorder than those without a mental disorder.[4] It should be noted that these characteristics also place individuals at risk for other psychiatric disorders, including posttraumatic stress disorder (PTSD) and major depressive disorder. To date, there has not been a well-designed study that clearly identifies predictors that

Table 1 Subtypes of adjustment disorder	
Subtype	Predominant Symptoms
Adjustment disorder with depressed mood	Low mood, tearfulness, or feelings of hopelessness
Adjustment disorder with anxiety	Nervousness, worry, jitteriness, or separation anxiety
Adjustment disorder with mixed anxiety and depressed mood	Combination of depression and anxiety
Adjustment disorder with disturbance of conduct	Disturbance of conduct
Adjustment disorder with mixed disturbance of emotions and conduct:	Both emotional symptoms (eg, depression, anxiety) and a disturbance of conduct
Adjustment disorder unspecified	Maladaptive reactions that are not classifiable as one of the specific subtypes of adjustment disorder

differentiate adjustment disorders from PTSD, depressive disorders, and anxiety disorders.[4]

The types of stressors that may lead to adjustment disorders include both traumatic events, such as exposure to actual or threatened death, as well as nontraumatic events such as interpersonal conflict, death of a loved one, unemployment, financial difficulties, or illness of a loved one or oneself.[3]

Prevalence

The prevalence of adjustment disorders in the general population ranges from 0.2% to 2.3%. Among those in a clinical setting, the prevalence of adjustment disorder is as high as 2.9%, indicating a higher prevalence in these populations as opposed to the general population.[1] The prevalence of adjustment disorders is also higher in populations that are undergoing stressful circumstances. For those living in a postconflict environment, the prevalence ranged from 6% to 40%.[5] For those who are unemployed, the prevalence is 27%,[6] and among those with a recent death in the family, the prevalence is 18%.[7] The prevalence of adjustment disorder is also higher than the general population in those who have a serious medical diagnosis (such as breast cancer), with rates ranging from 15% to 35%.[3]

Diagnosis

Although the current DSM V and ICD-11 diagnostic criteria of adjustment disorder states that other psychiatric disorders should not be present, adjustment disorder is often diagnosed in conjunction with major depressive disorder, generalized anxiety disorder, and posttraumatic stress disorder.[3] As a result, the separation of adjustment disorder is not as cleanly cut in clinic practice from other psychiatric diagnoses as these criteria would represent.

There is also concern that these diagnostic criteria may lead to a pathologizing of normal grief reactions or normal responses to stress. This concern exists since clinicians may simply check off the symptoms of adjustment disorder because it appears in the DSM V and ICD-11, rather than fully evaluating the individual patient in the context of his or her cultural norms.[2] Conversely, some are concerned that the loose definitions provided would result in an underdiagnosis of adjustment disorders, resulting in the delaying of much needed treatment of some patients.[2] The concerns about underdiagnosis are not only valid but concerning because there is an association of suicidality with adjustment disorder.[8]

The vague DSM V and ICD-11 criteria have also led to difficulty in researching the disorder and creating validated diagnostic tools. Several other tools have been researched as methods to diagnose adjustment disorder, such as the Hamilton Anxiety Rating Scale but are not validated to diagnose adjustment disorder.[9] As a result of this, the Adjustment Disorder New Module scale (ADNM-20) was created to assist clinicians with accurately diagnosing adjustment disorder.[10,11] Clinicians should be aware that this tool is based on the ICD-11 diagnostic criteria for adjustment disorder, not on the DSM V.[10] The ADNM-20 consists of 2 parts, a list of stressors and a list of symptoms, which include preoccupation, failure to adapt, depressive mood, avoidance, anxiety, and impulsivity.[10] The ADNM 20 has shown good reliability and internal consistency in research.[9,10] There is also a briefer assessment tool, the ADNM-8, which is shortened to 8 questions.[12] Both of these tools are still in development and require further research to back up their validity in clinical practice.

One of the key diagnostic features of adjustment disorder is an inciting stressor. If this stressor resolves, treatment may not be needed. However, there are reasons to consider treatment. These include shortening duration of distressing symptoms such as sleep impairment and anxiety, reducing chronic symptoms when the stressor is prolonged, enhancing resilience against recurring stressors, alleviating overwhelming and disabling symptoms affecting behaviors, and potentially preventing progression to major depression.[2]

Treatment

The treatment of choice for adjustment disorder is psychological therapy.[13] Initially, therapy methods that were effective in other psychiatric disorders (such as cognitive behavioral therapy and gestalt psychotherapy) were used with mixed results.[2] Therapy Program for Adjustment Disorders is one of the few therapies that is specifically for those with adjustment disorders. This is a problem-solving approach that can be used for both individuals and groups.[2] Self-directed and web-based therapies are being studied for adjustment disorder because the fluctuating nature of the symptoms requires highly accessible treatments.[9]

If patients do not respond to psychological therapy, pharmacotherapy can be considered. There are several herbal therapies that have been demonstrated as being useful in treating the anxiety subtype, including Kava Kava,[14] valerian,[15] and ginkgo biloba.[16] Several studies have also demonstrated that benzodiazepines are effective in reducing symptoms in adjustment disorder,[17] as is trazodone.[18] Trazodone has the added benefit of being lower risk for abuse or dependence.[19] The pharmacologic treatment with the best evidence for adjustment disorder is etifoxine,[20,21] although this drug is not Food and Drug Administration (FDA) approved.

SUMMARY

There are concerns that adjustment disorder might be pathologizing normal reactions to stressors. As in the case with EP above, the actions of the neighbor would cause anyone distress. This is where is the concept of adjustment disorder as the "mental flu"[1] likely originates. Many people will get the flu and most will recover. However, a small number of people with the flu will develop more serious symptoms and sequelae. This is similar to stress reactions: different individuals exposed to the same stressors will have different reactions. Some will have no issues, and some will develop an adjustment disorder. If these individuals have severe enough symptoms, they should be offered the option of either psychological or pharmacologic treatment. Adjustment disorder is also used at times as a precursor diagnosis for major depressive disorder and generalized anxiety disorder. If the patient's symptoms continue to persist beyond the removal of the stressor, one of these diagnoses should be considered.[1] There remain opportunities to more clearly define the diagnostic criteria, subtypes and stressors for adjustment disorder. Further research is also needed to identify a validated diagnostic tool and appropriate treatments.

CLINICS CARE POINTS

- Consider adjustment disorder as a diagnosis in patients who meet either the DSM V or ICD-11 diagnostic criteria.
- Adjustment disorder can present with either anxiety, depression, or a combination of these symptoms.
- Those with adjustment disorder should be offered either psychology therapy, pharmacotherapy or both, dependent on their needs.
- If a patient's symptoms continue beyond removal of the stressor, other psychiatric disorders should be considered.

DISCLOSURE

The author reports no financial conflicts of interest.

ACKNOWLEDGMENTS

Dr. Meagan Vermuelen support and assistance in the publication process.

REFERENCES

1. Zelviene P, Kazlauskas P. Adjustment Disorders: Current Perspectives. Neuropsych Dis Treat 2018;14:375–81.
2. Bachem R, Casey P. Adjustment Disorders: A Diagnosis whose time has come. J Affect Disord 2018;227:243–53.
3. O'Donnell ML, Agathos JA, Metcalf O, et al. Adjustment Disorders: Current Developments and Future Directions. Int J Environ Res Public Health 2019;16:2537.
4. Kelber MS, Morgan MA, Beech EH, et al. Systematic Review and meta-analysis of predictors for Adjustment Disorders in Adults. J Affect Disord 2022;304:43–58.
5. Dobricki M, Komproe IH, de Jong JTVM, et al. Adjustment disorders after severe life-events in four postconflict settings. Soc Psychiatry Psychiatr Epidemiol 2010; 45:39–46.
6. Perkonigg A, Lorenz L, Maercker A. Prevalence and correlates of ICD-11 adjustment disorder: Findings from the Zurich Adjustment Disorder Study. Int J Clin Health Psychol 2018;18:209–17.
7. Killikelly C, Lorenz L, Bauer S, et al. Prolonged grief disorder: Its co-occurrence with adjustment disorder and post-traumatic stress disorder in a bereaved Israeli general-population sample. J Affect Disord 2019;249:307–14.
8. Casey P, Jabbar F, O'Leary E, et al. Suicidal behaviours in adjustment disorder and depressive episode. J Affect Disord 2015;174:441–6.

9. Bachem R, Perkonigg A, Stein DJ, et al. Measuring the ICD-11 adjustment disorder concept: validity and sensitivity to change of the adjustment disorder – new module questionnaire in a clinical interven tion study. Int J Methods Psychiatr Res 2017;26(4):1–9.

10. Einsle F, Köllner V, Dannemann S, et al. Development and validation of a self-report for the assessment of adjustment disorders. Psychol Health Med 2010; 15(5):584–95.

11. Lorenz L, Bachem RC, Maercker A. The adjustment disorder-new module 20 as a screening instrument: cluster analysis and cut-off values. Int J Occup Environ Med 2016;7(4):215–20.

12. Eimontas J, Gegieckaite G, Dovydaitiene M, et al. The role of therapist support on effectiveness of an internet-based modular self-help inter vention for adjustment disorder: a randomized controlled trial. Anxiety Stress Coping 2017;31(2): 146–58.

13. Strain J, Friedman MJ. Considering adjustment disorders as stress response syndromes for DSM-5. Depress Anxiety 2011;28:818–23.

14. Volz HP, Kieser M. Kava-kava extract WS 1490 versus placebo in anxiety dis or-ders. A randomized placebo-controlled 25-week outpatient trial. Pharmacopsychiatry 1997;30:1–5.

15. Bourin M, Bougerol T, Guitton B, et al. A combination of plant extracts in the treatment of outpatients with adjustment disorder with anxious mood: controlled study versus placebo. Fundam Clin Pharmacol 1997;11:127–32.

16. Woelk H, Arnoldt KH, Kieser M, et al. Ginkgo biloba special extract EGb 761 in generalized anxiety disorder and adjustment disorder with anxious mood: a randomized, double-blind, placebo-controlled trial. J Psychiatr Res 2007;41:472–80.

17. Ansseau M, Bataille M, Briole G, et al. Controlled comparison of tianeptine, alprazolam and mianserin in the treatment of adjustment disorders with anxiety and depression. Hum Psychopharmacol Clin Exp 1996;11(4):293–8.

18. Razavi D, Kormoss N, Collard A, et al. Comparative study of the efficacy and safety of trazodone versus clorazepate in the treatment of adjustment disorders in cancer patients: a pilot study. J Int Med Res 1999;27:264–72.

19. Constantin D, Dinu EA, Rogozea L. Therapeutic Interventions for Adjustment Disorder: A Systematic Review. Am J Ther 2020;27:375–86.

20. Nguyen N, Fakra E, Pradel V, et al. Efficacy of etifoxine compared to lorazepam monotherapy in the treatment of patients with adjustment disorders with anxiety: a double-blind controlled study in general practice. Hum Psychopharmacol Clin Exp 2006;21:139–49.

21. Stein DJ. Etifoxine versus alprazolam for the treatment of adjustment disorder with anxiety: a randomized controlled trial. Adv Ther 2015;3:57–68.

Person-First Treatment Strategies

Weight Bias and Impact on Mental Health of People Living with Obesity

Nina Crowley, PhD, RD*

KEYWORDS

- Obesity • Weight bias • Stigma • Person-first language • Mental health

KEY POINTS

- Internalizing weight bias significantly and independently contributes to poor emotional health beyond the impact of body mass index (BMI) or excess weight.
- Health care providers can be inadvertently contributing to further bias and health care avoidance among their patients if they are not aware of subtle ways their communication and language can stigmatize.
- Person-first language is one of many strategies to show respect for patients and build a trusting relationship that will promote adherence to treatment and better outcomes for both patient and provider.
- Weight bias can be measured and there are strategies to reduce its impact through assessment, education, communication strategies, language choice, intentional clinical environment design, and advocacy.

INTRODUCTION
Nature of the Problem: Obesity and Weight Stigma

At this point in time, most Americans are carrying excess weight and are considered as having the chronic disease of obesity or pre-obesity/overweight and are at risk for development of weight-related health problems such as type 2 diabetes and cardiovascular disease. Despite associations with morbidity, mortality, and psychosocial implications, our society has not yet addressed treatment or prevention from a systemic perspective. From a public health perspective, it is perplexing to have a majority living with a chronic health condition and have minimal commitment to prevention, treatment, or policy addressing the condition. Paradoxically, people who have obesity are also likely to internalize weight bias and harbor bias toward other people with the same condition.

Medical Body Composition for Seca Corporation
* 1463 Longpsur Drive, Mt Pleasant, SC 29466.
E-mail address: ninamcrowley@gmail.com

Prim Care Clin Office Pract 50 (2023) 89–101
https://doi.org/10.1016/j.pop.2022.10.002
primarycare.theclinics.com

Weight bias involves having negative attitudes toward people perceived to have the visible characteristic of excess weight.[1] Negative views lead to discrimination and poor treatment in a variety of areas for people with obesity. Bias can be considered explicit when these attitudes are within one's consciousness and accessible to the person who could both report and control their views, such as sneering remarks or "fat jokes."[2] Implicit attitudes refer to the automatic reactions that occur when encountering a stimulus, in this case, someone perceived as carrying excess weight.[3] An important distinction between explicit and implicit attitudes is that implicit attitudes are activated even if the person considers the evaluation or attitude to be in line with their personal beliefs.[4] Explicit beliefs are more of an evaluation or judgment after reflection and assessment of the object and can be considered a personal belief one believes to be true.[5]

Implicit bias has received much attention as these "default" attitudes predict behaviors that are beyond conscious control.[3] Like racism, explicit attitudes are direct and overtly expressed and implicit are indirect and subtle. Unlike racism, there seems to be less normative pressure to suppress attitudes toward people with obesity, and it has been considered the "last socially acceptable form of prejudice or discrimination."[3] It has been estimated that 40% of adults have been a target of weight-based teasing, unfair treatment, or discrimination.[6,7] Although implicit attitudes were once defined as stable and resistant to change, there has been more evidence that these automatic affective reactions can be influenced by context and can be modified.[8]

Bias toward people with obesity is rooted in the pervasive belief that body weight is within a person's control and that people who are not able to "control" their weight are lazy, gluttonous, or weak.[1] A shocking 59% of Americans believe that obesity is caused by a lack of willpower.[9] Like the addiction model, being unable to control your "affliction" is considered "irresponsible" and a sign of a moral failure and therefore a target of moral failure.[10] The traditional American value of self-determinism and individualism where people "get what they deserve" and are responsible for their life situation combined with the cultural view that to lose weight, one should simply "eat less, move more" allow weight stigma to thrive.[11] The more that a disease is perceived as being under a person's volitional control, the more emotional the response like stigmatized attitudes and behavioral consequences like discrimination will co-occur.[12]

INTERNALIZED WEIGHT STIGMA

Internalized weight bias begins when someone becomes aware that they are devalued by others in society.[12] These negative attitudes or stereotypes may be endorsed by a person at a higher weight and applied to oneself. This can be seen when people blame themselves for their "lack of control" and believe that they are "just lazy and lack motivation to change." Internalization of these negative stereotypes can lead to lower self-esteem, low self-worth, and self-devaluation.[13] Patients may state that they have daily feelings about being "disappointed in self," that it is "their own fault," they may feel "like a failure," or even "ugly and disgusting."

Interestingly, weight bias internalization significantly and independently contributes to poor emotional health beyond the impact of BMI or excess weight.[14] Weight bias associated with obesity may also pose a greater threat to an individual's health than increasing BMI.[15] Studies have associated internalized weight bias with depression, anxiety, stress, clinical eating pathology, binge eating, health-related quality of life, and poor weight loss maintenance.[7] Owing to the cycle of low self-efficacy and feeling capable of doing what they feel they "should" be doing, they may overeat, avoid activity, and give up hope, resulting in feeling sad, guilty, ashamed, and frustrated, which continues to perpetuate this cycle.[16]

MEASURING WEIGHT BIAS

Understanding weight bias and obesity stigma requires knowledge of how it is assessed. Many of the currently available measures use adjective check lists with a rating scale for characteristics attributed to people with "thin" or "fat" body size. Implicit-association tests (IATs) are available as self-report tests for individuals to measure their own implicit weight bias.[2] IATs are timed word association tests where you are given words that fit into one of the four categories. People find it easier to categorize words faster when the pair matches their attitude than when it is mismatched, thereby finishing the tasks faster. People with greater levels of bias pair more words in the time allotted when "fat people" is paired with negative characteristics (slow, lazy, sluggish) than positive characteristics (determined, motivated, eager). The latency of time taken to respond to positive or negative attributes dictates scores and strong preferences to body types that are either "thin" or "fat."[17]

Other validated measures for assessment of weight bias and obesity stigma include:

- Anti-fat Attitudes Questionnaire[18]
- Anti-fat Attitudes Scale[19]
- Anti-fat Attitudes Test[20]
- Attitudes Toward Obese Persons and Beliefs About Obese Persons scales[21]
- Fat Phobia Scale[22]
- Obese Persons Traits Survey[23]
- Universal Measure of Bias–Fat[24]
- Weight Bias Internalization Scale[25]

Prevalence of Weight Bias

For people living with obesity, the relationship with their health care providers is of the utmost importance. Seeking advice from a provider requires a supportive relationship built on trust. Although most providers are committed to proving the best care and not intentionally harming their patients, implicit or unintentional weight bias can get in the way.[26] Research shows that health care providers hold biased attitudes about people living with obesity that most certainly can get in the way of providing patient-centered care and helping patients achieve their best outcomes.[27]

Weight bias has been reported in physicians, nurses, dietitians, exercise therapists, psychologists, and exercise professionals and is as pervasive as it is in the general population.[28] Strong bias is found in nearly all types of health care providers and has a negative impact on their ability to provide medical services for those who are already impacted by the chronic disease of obesity.[29]

Bias toward individuals with obesity starts early on as professionals, in college health profession majors, 93% view people with obesity as lazy, short on willpower, lacking endurance, overeating, self-indulgent and weak.[17,30] In a study of more than 2500 US adults with overweight/obesity, approximately 70% of participants reported experiencing weight stigma from a doctor, and more than half reported that this happened more than once.[31]

Explicit, negative attitudes are captured by responses of health care professionals who express negative feelings toward people with obesity, such as considering them as "unmotivated" or "unlikely to adhere to treatment recommendations." Weight bias may be expressed by health care providers through contemptuous, patronizing, and disrespectful treatment.[32] Attributing all a patient's health issues to their excess body weight can also directly contribute to the weight stigma that patients experience.

If education about obesity as a disease state was enough to eliminate bias, our health care providers and those specializing in obesity as a disease state would not experience in biased attitudes and behaviors. There is a continued need for health care professionals to become aware of bias as a first step to counteract it. Some of the discrepancy in provision of appropriate care for obesity comes from the lack of understanding and knowledge about obesity treatment guidelines. Incorporation of the most evidence-based approaches for management of obesity has not been widely included in primary care practices or formal education pathways.[33–35]

As a result, fewer than 5% of individuals are treated with the current effective nutritional, behavioral, medical, and surgical modalities available.[36] Providers report significant obstacles to obesity counseling such as the discomfort of opening a conversation, lack of time to provide appropriate counseling, and insufficient training in nutrition and obesity treatment guidelines.[37] One study showed that 94% of internal medicine residents believed it was their role to discuss nutrition with patients, and only 14% believed adequately trained in counseling.[38] In addition, the added barriers of limited reimbursement and inadequate access to care for the spectrum of treatment modalities make treatment planning difficult.

Consequences of Weight Bias for Health Care Providers

A longitudinal study shows that those who experience weight discrimination have a 60% increased risk of death, irrespective of their weight.[39] In addition, weight bias and stigma are considered psychosocial contributors to the epidemic rates of obesity.[16] Not only is there a need to better treat the disease of obesity, but there is also a clear need to address the consequences that people with obesity experience because of internalized weight bias.

Although weight bias and stigma have negative consequences in families, workplaces, education, and the media, its prevalence in health care providers seems to be the most alarming given our role in helping people improve their health. Patients who believe judged or stigmatized when they interact with their provider are less likely to return to preventive care visits.[40] Patients with obesity perceive their physicians as spending less time discussing and educating them about their health and treatment options.[41] Providers may use less patient-centered communication when providers make judgments that the patients are unlikely to follow through with the recommendations. Patients also believe their doctors are unable to appreciate challenges they face.

Negative attitudes held by health care providers influence the way they connect with their patients and have serious consequences for the clinical treatment of people with obesity. Health care providers have been found to spend less time with people with obesity, discuss treatment options less often, and limit communication about obesity as well as view their patients as unwilling to engage in weight management.[42]

Often, there is a mismatch of provider and patient's variable understanding of motivation for change. Owing to internalized weight bias, patients often think that it is their "personal responsibility" to manage their own weight, and do not consider it a medical issue. Many providers consider perceived patient lack of motivation as a barrier to even bringing up the discussion with them to discuss treatment options and lack of adherence to a plan a compliance or adherence issue.[43] Meanwhile, patients who experience and internalize stigma from their provider are less likely to follow a recommended eating plan.[44] However, a recent study found that diagnosis and discussion about weight management with the provider is more likely to result in patient's engaging in weight management efforts.[45]

The longer someone avoids treatment out of fear of the way they might be judged, the greater the likelihood of symptoms progressing to medical conditions in which care is more involved and expensive.[46]

Mental Health Consequences

Experiences and internalization of weight bias and stigma are robustly associated with poor mental health outcomes. As compared with those who have not experienced discrimination due to weight, those who have experienced weight stigma have two-fold greater odds for having depression and anxiety.[13,47] Internalized weight bias is associated with decreased self-esteem, poor body image, and body dissatisfaction.[31,48] Internalizing weight bias is related to greater rates of binge eating, dietary restraint, emotional eating, weight cycling, and more symptoms of food addiction.[13] Tomiyama suggests that stigma leads to weight gain through a feedback loop model where weight stigma is a stressor leading to increased cortisol levels and increased food intake, unhealthy eating and weight-control behaviors, binge eating, emotional eating, and further weight gain, which provokes further stigma.[49,50]

Even when controlling for BMI and general life stress, associations between stigma and mental health remain strong, further highlighting the unique contribution to psychological distress.[48] Both experiences and internalization of weight stigma have been found to mediate the relationship between BMI and psychological outcomes, suggesting that stigma plays a prominent role in explaining the relationship between obesity and mental health.[13]

STRATEGIES TO COMBAT WEIGHT BIAS IN PRACTICE
Awareness and Education on Complex Nature of Obesity

One of the most effective ways to reduce weight bias in health care providers may be to increase education of obesity as a disease.[51] Formal education should not reinforce existing biases and opinions about the personal responsibility for obesity. Weight bias can also be reduced when providers move focus away from body weight and turn to the health conditions for which obesity is a risk factor and can be targeted. Having causal beliefs such as that lack of self-discipline or poor eating habits lead to obesity are related to increased stereotyping and stigma, whereas a focus on genetic, metabolic, environmental causes is related to reduced stigma.[13] The understanding of the complex etiology of obesity helps providers communicate about many factors related to predisposition to obesity and reduces self-blaming for not being able to overcome challenges. Understanding that the heritability index of obesity is 40% to 70%, similar to a person's height, is critical in being able to understand the disease and empathize with patients who feel blamed for their size.[52]

Integrating sensitive communication training during tertiary education, to ensure that future health care provider (HCPs) develop greater awareness and understanding of the potential influence of weight bias on their provision of care and how weight bias may negatively influence the patient–provider relationship as well as patient outcomes[53] is an opportunity to help reshape the future of obesity care. The American Society for Metabolic and Bariatric Surgery (ASMBS) position statement on weight bias and stigma recommends obesity medicine as part of medical training with a focus on increasing knowledge, competency, sensitive communication, and confidence in treating patients with obesity. They suggest that there is a need for greater guidance on how to raise the topic of weight loss in a non-stigmatizing manner and provide recommendations that are relevant, evidence-based, individualized, and realistic.[54]

Personal biases can unintentionally harm the relationship between the provider and patient. Increased awareness of one's own personal assumptions, attitudes, or believes about weight and health can impact eye contact, body language, tone of voice, facial expressions, nonverbal gestures, and special distance between people.[55] Providers should challenge the conventional views that attribute the cause of obesity to sedentary lifestyle and consider evidence indicating contributions of genetic, epigenetic, foodborne, sleep, circadian dysrhythmia, psychological stress, endocrine disruptor, medication, intrauterine, and intergenerational effects.[56]

Awareness may begin from didactic learning or taking individual IAT to objectively assess implicit bias that may not be within awareness of the provider.[57] A few studies have examined traditional classroom and web-based educational curricula using instruction about causes of obesity, awareness of weight bias impact on practice, and sensitivity training with short-term effectiveness for improving explicit and implicit attitudes.[58] Others have used media-based weight bias reduction interventions with videos, audio recordings, and role-playing, which have shown promise in reducing explicit bias and increasing empathy, although not implicit bias.[59] More recent studies have looked at experiential learning such as witnessing treatments recommended for patients with obesity, interacting with patients, and working with experts in the field.[41] Exposing students to obesity treatments where they try the diet that patients are being asked to follow or work with bariatric patients preparing for surgery may decrease negative attitudes.[59] Multicomponent programs with multifaceted content seem to be most effective.

Communication and Language

Word choice is very important when communicating to patients about their weight and health risk. An effective way to reduce bias is by considering a shift to language used with patients. Like the shift in language that has been used for "people with disabilities" for years, people-first language for people with obesity has become standard in the medical obesity care community. People-first language refers to not labeling people by the disease they have. People should be considered as whole people, not a diagnosis or an "obese person," but a "person with the disease of obesity." Instead of labeling the person as their disease, consider using "patient/individual/person with obesity" or even "person living with obesity" or "person in a larger body."[60] This language choice acknowledges respect and dignity toward the person and can start a conversation off on the right foot.

Some of the most stigmatizing words that communicate blame about one's size are Fat, Morbidly Obese, Obese, Heavy, Chubby, and Extremely Obese.[61] Less stigmatizing words include Weight, BMI if explained properly, Weight Problem, Unhealthy Weight, and Overweight. In a recent systematic review examining people's perceptions of and preferences for weight-related terminology, there was a preference for more neutral terms (weight, unhealthy weight, "your weight may be damaging your health") and unacceptance for terms such as obese/obesity and fat/fatness.[60] The term BMI had mixed findings from being preferred to not being desirable or motivating.

Just like it has become common practice to ask people what pronouns they prefer to use for gender orientation, people have differing preferences on what words they prefer that you use when referring to their weight. Some have reclaimed the use of "fat" and prefer this to be used. Health care professionals do not have to know the "best" term if they approach from a place of curiosity and ask patients directly. Consider using neutral terminology and saying, "Could we talk about your weight today?" and acknowledge that people have different preferences regarding terms, and then ask which would make them feel most comfortable.[13]

The way in which health care providers discuss eating habits, physical activity, and health behaviors can be another way that providers are unintentionally stigmatizing. The STOP Obesity Alliance guide recommends a modified approach to the "5 As" model for weight management counseling in primary care with the addition of "Ask."[62] This model has been helpful in teaching providers to listen first before giving advice, becoming more patient-centered, and helping patients feel more motivated and have stronger intentions to change behavior.[63]

- *Ask* permission to discuss weight and health
  - "Is now a good time for us to discuss how your weight and health may be affecting each other and how we can work together on it?"
  - "I am concerned about how your weight may be affecting your health. Today there are many effective treatments for obesity"
  - Ask what terms they would prefer you use to discuss their weight
  - Listen and acknowledge their concerns
- *Assess* obesity-related clinical status
  - Assess patient's desired weight loss goal and reasons for wanting to lose weight
  - Refer to prescreen data: BMI, weight history, diet history, medications, physical activities, comorbidities, risk factors, stress, sleep, quality of life, and mental health
  - Refer to blood tests, comorbidities, weight history/trajectory, and obesity-focused physical assessment
- *Advise* on health risks, benefits, options
  - Focus on positive aspects of health improvement, follow USPSTF guidelines to offer intensive, multicomponent behavioral interventions
  - Convey the challenge of weight management and potential for weight cycling
  - Use shared decision-making to establish next steps
- *Agree* regarding treatment goals and plans
  - Establish trust and shared decision-making
  - Agree on weight loss, lifestyle, and behavioral goals, if not met, consider escalating intervention or adjusting treatment goals
  - Recommendations may differ depending on cultural background
  - Collaborate using SMART goals and discuss effectiveness of treatment modalities
- *Assist* with barriers, resources, providers, and follow-up
  - Assist patient by creating a plan and document to communicate with rest of team
  - Leverage the entire care team and discus referrals to registered dietitian nutritionists, behavioral health providers, certified obesity medicine providers
- *Arrange* for follow-up
  - Arrange for patient to have resources, close follow-up, and coordination of care

Obesity, weight, and health are intensely personal subjects, and different people have different issues as well as different goals. The use of patient-centered care is critical to facilitate conversations regarding weight management. Providers can initiate a collaborative conversation about obesity and can use shared decision-making to build trust and guide treatment options. When there is a choice to be made between options, providers can guide patients to discuss benefits and harms of the options while keeping a focus on what is important to the patient. Evidence-based practice includes a focus on the patient's perspective, experience, and feelings about past attempts at

Table 1
Weight bias/obesity stigma resources

Resource	Weblink
ASMBS Position Statement on Weight Bias and Stigma[54]	https://link.springer.com/article/10.1007/s11695-020-04525-0
Canadian Obesity Network image bank	http://www.obesitynetwork.ca/images-bank
European Association for the Study of Obesity image bank	http://easo.org/media-portal/obesity-image-bank/
Examine explicit and implicit bias with IAT	http://www.implicit.harvard.edu
Guidelines for Media Portrayals of Individuals Affected by Obesity	https://www.obesityaction.org/action-through-advocacy/weight-bias/media-guidelines-for-obesity/
Joint international consensus statement for ending stigma of obesity[56]	https://www.soard.org/article/S1550-7289(19)30168-6/fulltext
Obesity Action Coalition Weight Bias Resources	https://www.obesityaction.org/action-through-advocacy/weight-bias/weight-bias-resources/
Obesity Action Coalition Image Library	https://www.obesityaction.org/get-educated/public-resources/oac-image-gallery/
Provider Competencies for the Prevention and Management of Obesity	https://www.obesitycompetencies.gwu.edu/competencies
Strategies to Overcome and Prevent Obesity Alliance: Why Weight Guide	http://whyweightguide.org/
University of Connecticut Rudd Center Library Images/Media Gallery	https://uconnruddcenter.org/media-gallery/#
World Obesity Federation image bank	http://www.imagebank.worldobesity.org/

weight changes and approaches they have tried. Goal setting should be driven by the patient's individual health goals, and not what the provider feels the patient "should" be doing.

Education materials are important to consider within this framework as well. Creating interactive education materials in collaboration with people who have had the lived experience of obesity can help to reduce stigma.[64] In addition, it is advised to use real patients whenever possible to accurately capture the patient experience and provide feedback to providers about how patients experience provider bias. Several resources are provided for image banks for use in presentations and social media to portray patients positively and engaging in activities to avoid further stigma and alienating people with obesity (**Table 1**).

Clinical Environment

Creating a comfortable clinical environment that is appropriate for patients of all body sizes is an integral part of reducing weight stigma. Demonstrating respect for people living in a larger body means ensuring that the office has seating, restrooms, examination rooms, tables, scales, blood pressure cuffs, and gowns that accommodate their size. Scales that have a wide platform with handles for support and that are situated in a physical area that offers privacy is important.

Images of individuals with obesity are common sources of stigma, and derogatory images used in the context of trying to help people with their health may, in fact, perpetuate further bias. There are several organizations that have worked to create image banks for professionals to use in their presentations, on Web sites, and in social media so that people with obesity are portrayed as whole people, and not "headless," or taking a bite from fast food (see **Table 1**).

Patients see their primary care provider for many reasons, and some acute care issues may not be appropriate times to weigh or even discuss weight. Other times, there may not be enough time at a visit where discussion of weight is appropriate. Using an approach based in genuine curiosity, consider asking the patient, "Is there a future time that might be appropriate for us to discuss how your weight and health may be affecting each other and how we might work together to address it?"[62]

Policy Approaches

Although individual-level approaches are often the first step in addressing assumptions and reducing stigma, Alberga and colleagues[65] argue for an upstream, population-level approach. Suggestions include legislation to prohibit weight discrimination, mandatory curriculum to train health care professionals, employment and health care policies, financial incentives for avoiding bias and stigma, stringent media guidelines, and modifying the built environment to accommodate people of all sizes. This comprehensive approach offers a map toward a future where weight bias is both unacceptable and not tolerated.

SUMMARY

Ignorance of the consequences of weight bias on individuals in larger bodies is no longer an option. People with obesity are experiencing negative health outcomes, not just from carrying excess weight or risk for other chronic disease, but from internalizing the bias and stigma that they experience. Internalized weight bias can be more deleterious to mental health than the excess weight that someone is being stigmatized for. Health risks from obesity are serious and people with obesity need appropriate care from their health care team, however, if the health care providers are perpetuating the bias and stigma, they are exacerbating the problem. Individual providers can take action to learn more about their own biases, and how to work to reduce it. Patients who trust and feel comfortable with their providers will be more likely to return to care and engage in the therapeutic goal setting if they do not believe judged by their provider. Paying attention to communication style, language around weight, health and obesity, and continuing to learn about the complex disease state can help. Just like the disease itself, weight bias reduction is complex and will require a multifaceted solution with effort from advocates from all areas of the system.

CLINICS CARE POINTS

- Integrate education about the complex disease of obesity, heritability, and effective interventions into medical school training and clinical care at every level of education.

- Take and implicit-association test to assess your own personal levels of bias and identify areas that require further work and training.

- Review people-first language and enlist colleagues to help ensure you are working to use this in all patient encounters, conversations with providers and in presentations and scholarly writing.

- Consider terms you use to discuss weight, health, and obesity with patients and practice asking patients what words they prefer.

- Practice using the "5 As" model with patients to improve encounters when discussing their weight.
- Review patient-facing materials and enlist help from people with obesity to provide perspective on all aspects of education and communication.
- Create comfortable clinical environments for people in larger bodies and consider seating, restrooms, examination rooms, tables, scales, blood pressure cuffs, and gowns that accommodate their size.
- Use resources available for appropriate images of people with obesity for use at all levels of practice from patient-facing materials to Web marketing to social media and professional presentations
- Do not stop with your individual practice or your clinic; advocate for patient-centered care, appropriate language, and access to care for people with obesity at all levels.

DISCLOSURE

The author works for seca corporation, but this work has no impact on the content of this article.

REFERENCES

1. Puhl RM, Brownell KD. Psychosocial origins of obesity stigma: toward changing a powerful and pervasive bias. Obes Rev 2003;4(4):213–27.
2. Greenwald AG, McGhee DE, Schwartz JL. Measuring individual differences in implicit cognition: the implicit association test. J Pers Soc Psychol 1998;74(6):1464.
3. Watts K, Cranney J. The nature and implications of implicit weight bias. Curr Psychiatry Rev 2009;5(2):110–26.
4. Devine PG. Stereotypes and prejudice: their automatic and controlled components. J Pers Soc Psychol 1989;56(1):5.
5. Gawronski B, Bodenhausen GV. Associative and propositional processes in evaluation: an integrative review of implicit and explicit attitude change. Psychol Bull 2006;132(5):692.
6. Puhl RM, Latner JD, O'Brien K, et al. A multinational examination of weight bias: predictors of anti-fat attitudes across four countries. Int J Obes 2015;39(7):1166–73.
7. Himmelstein MS, Puhl RM, Quinn DM. Intersectionality: an understudied framework for addressing weight stigma. Am J Prev Med 2017;53(4):421–31.
8. Blair IV. The malleability of automatic stereotypes and prejudice. Personal Social Psychol Rev 2002;6(3):242–61.
9. Taylor P, Funk C, Craighill P. Americans see weight problems everywhere but in the mirror. Philadelphia: Pew Foundation Social Trends Report; 2006.
10. Crandall CS, Reser AH. Attributions and weight-based prejudice. In: Brownell KD, Puhl RM, Schwartz MB, et al, editors. Weight bias: nature, consequences, and remedies. New York: Guilford Publications; 2005. p. 83–96.
11. Crandall CS, Martinez R. Culture, ideology, and antifat attitudes. Pers Soc Psychol Bull 1996;22(11):1165–76.
12. Corrigan P, Markowitz FE, Watson A, et al. An attribution model of public discrimination towards persons with mental illness. J Health Soc Behav 2003;44(2):162–79.

13. Pearl RL, Puhl RM. Weight bias internalization and health: a systematic review. Obes Rev 2018;19(8):1141–63.

14. Carels RA, Burmeister J, Oehlhof MW, et al. Internalized weight bias: ratings of the self, normal weight, and obese individuals and psychological maladjustment. J Behav Med 2013;36(1):86–94.

15. Tomiyama AJ, Carr D, Granberg EM, et al. How and why weight stigma drives the obesity 'epidemic'and harms health. BMC Med 2018;16(1):1–6.

16. Pearl RL, Puhl RM, Himmelstein MS, et al. Weight stigma and weight-related health: associations of self-report measures among adults in weight management. Ann Behav Med 2020;54(11):904–14.

17. Blanton C, Brooks JK, McKnight L. Weight bias in university health professions students. J Allied Health 2016;45(3):212–8.

18. Crandall CS. Prejudice against fat people: ideology and self-interest. J Pers Soc Psychol 1994;66(5):882.

19. Morrison TG, O'connor WE. Psychometric properties of a scale measuring negative attitudes toward overweight individuals. J Soc Psychol 1999;139(4):436–45.

20. Lewis RJ, Cash TF, Bubb-Lewis C. Prejudice toward fat people: the development and validation of the antifat attitudes test. Obes Res 1997;5(4):297–307.

21. Allison DB, Basile VC, Yuker HE. The measurement of attitudes toward and beliefs about obese persons. Int J Eat Disord 1991;10(5):599–607.

22. Robinson BBE, Bacon LC, O'reilly J. Fat phobia: Measuring, understanding, and changing anti-fat attitudes. Int J Eat Disord 1993;14(4):467–80.

23. Puhl RM, Schwartz MB, Brownell KD. Impact of perceived consensus on stereotypes about obese people: a new approach for reducing bias. Health Psychol 2005;24(5):517.

24. Latner JD, O'Brien KS, Durso LE, et al. Weighing obesity stigma: the relative strength of different forms of bias. Int J Obes 2008;32(7):1145–52.

25. Durso LE, Latner JD. Understanding self-directed stigma: development of the weight bias internalization scale. Obesity 2008;16(S2):S80–6.

26. Lawrence BJ, Kerr D, Pollard CM, et al. Weight bias among health care professionals: A systematic review and meta-analysis. Obesity 2021;29(11):1802–12.

27. Joseph-Williams N, Edwards A, Elwyn G. Power imbalance prevents shared decision making. BMJ 2014;348:3178–80.

28. Sabin JA, Marini M, Nosek BA. Implicit and explicit anti-fat bias among a large sample of medical doctors by BMI, race/ethnicity and gender. PLoS One 2012; 7(11):e48448.

29. Fruh SM, Nadglowski J, Hall HR, et al. Obesity stigma and bias. J Nurse Pract 2016;12(7):425–32.

30. Jung FU, Luck-Sikorski C, Wiemers N, et al. Dietitians and nutritionists: stigma in the context of obesity. A systematic review. PLoS One 2015;10(10):e0140276.

31. Puhl RM, Brownell KD. Confronting and coping with weight stigma: an investigation of overweight and obese adults. Obesity 2006;14(10):1802–15.

32. Alberga AS, Edache IY, Forhan M, et al. Weight bias and health care utilization: a scoping review, . Primary Health Care Research & Development. United Kingdom: Cambridge University Press; 2019. p. 20.

33. Butsch WS, Kushner RF, Alford S, et al. Low priority of obesity education leads to lack of medical students' preparedness to effectively treat patients with obesity: results from the US medical school obesity education curriculum benchmark study. BMC Med Educ 2020;20(1):1–6.

34. Kushner RF, Horn DB, Butsch WS, et al. Development of obesity competencies for medical education: a report from the Obesity Medicine Education Collaborative. Obesity 2019;27(7):1063–7.
35. Bradley DW, Dietz WH. Provider competencies for the prevention and management of obesity. Washington, DC: Bipartisan Policy Center; 2017.
36. Dietz WH, Baur LA, Hall K, et al. Management of obesity: improvement of health-care training and systems for prevention and care. The Lancet 2015;385(9986): 2521–33.
37. Mastrocola MR, Roque SS, Benning LV, et al. Obesity education in medical schools, residencies, and fellowships throughout the world: a systematic review. Int J Obes 2020;44(2):269–79.
38. Vetter ML, Herring SJ, Sood M, et al. What do resident physicians know about nutrition? An evaluation of attitudes, self-perceived proficiency and knowledge. J Am Coll Nutr 2008;27(2):287–98.
39. Sutin AR, Stephan Y, Terracciano A. Weight discrimination and risk of mortality. Psychol Sci 2015;26(11):1803–11.
40. Puhl RM, Heuer CA. The stigma of obesity: a review and update. Obesity 2009; 17(5):941.
41. Phelan SM, Burgess DJ, Yeazel MW, et al. Impact of weight bias and stigma on quality of care and outcomes for patients with obesity. Obes Rev 2015;16(4): 319–26.
42. Mold F, Forbes A. Patients' and professionals' experiences and perspectives of obesity in health-care settings: a synthesis of current research. Health Expect 2013;16(2):119–42.
43. Kaplan LM, Golden A, Jinnett K, et al. Perceptions of barriers to effective obesity care: results from the national ACTION study. Obesity 2018;26(1):61–9.
44. Raves DM, Brewis A, Trainer S, et al. Bariatric surgery patients' perceptions of weight-related stigma in healthcare settings impair post-surgery dietary adherence. Front Psychol 2016;7:1497.
45. Ciemins EL, Casanova D. Obesity care management collaborative. Washington, D.C: Lecture presented at: STOP Obesity Roundtable; 2019.
46. Schwartz MB, Chambliss HON, Brownell KD, et al. Weight bias among health professionals specializing in obesity. Obes Res 2003;11(9):1033–9.
47. Hatzenbuehler ML, Keyes KM, Hasin DS. Associations between perceived weight discrimination and the prevalence of psychiatric disorders in the general population. Obesity 2009;17(11):2033–9.
48. Papadopoulos S, Brennan L. Correlates of weight stigma in adults with overweight and obesity: a systematic literature review. Obesity 2015;23(9):1743–60.
49. Tomiyama AJ. Weight stigma is stressful. A review of evidence for the Cyclic Obesity/Weight-Based Stigma model. Appetite 2014;82:8–15.
50. Puhl RM, King KM. Weight discrimination and bullying. Best Pract Res Clin Endocrinol Metab 2013;27(2):117–27.
51. Poustchi Y, Saks NS, Piasecki AK, et al. Brief intervention effective in reducing weight bias in medical students. Fam Med 2013;45(5):345.
52. Herrera BM, Lindgren CM. The genetics of obesity. Curr Diab Rep 2010;10(6): 498–505.
53. Kushner RF, Zeiss DM, Feinglass JM, et al. An obesity educational intervention for medical students addressing weight bias and communication skills using standardized patients. BMC Med Educ 2014;14(1):1–8.
54. Eisenberg D, Noria S, Grover B, et al. ASMBS position statement on weight bias and stigma. Surg Obes Relat Dis 2019;15(6):814–21.

55. Pont SJ, Puhl R, Cook SR, et al. Stigma experienced by children and adolescents with obesity. Pediatrics 2017;140(6).
56. Rubino F, Puhl RM, Cummings DE, et al. Joint international consensus statement for ending stigma of obesity. Nat Med 2020;26(4):485–97.
57. Gudzune KA, Bennett WL, Cooper LA, et al. Patients who feel judged about their weight have lower trust in their primary care providers. Patient Educ Couns 2014; 97(1):128–31.
58. Doshi RS, Gudzune KA. Clinical practices to mitigate weight bias. Bariatric Times 2018;15(4):12–6.
59. Swift JA, Tischler V, Markham S, et al. Are anti-stigma films a useful strategy for reducing weight bias among trainee healthcare professionals? Results of a pilot randomized control trial. Obes Facts 2013;6(1):91–102.
60. Puhl RM. What words should we use to talk about weight? A systematic review of quantitative and qualitative studies examining preferences for weight-related terminology. Obes Rev 2020;21(6):e13008.
61. Puhl R, Peterson JL, Luedicke J. Fighting obesity or obese persons? Public perceptions of obesity-related health messages. Int J Obes 2013;37(6):774–82.
62. Gallagher C, Corl A, Dietz WH, et al. Weight can't wait: a guide to discussing obesity and organizing treatment in the primary care setting. Obesity 2021; 29(5):821–4.
63. Tucker S, Bramante C, Conroy M, et al. The most undertreated chronic disease: addressing obesity in primary care settings. Curr Obes Rep 2021;10(3):396–408.
64. Nyblade L, Stockton MA, Giger K, et al. Stigma in health facilities: why it matters and how we can change it. BMC Med 2019;17(1):1–15.
65. Alberga AS, Russell-Mayhew S, von Ranson KM, et al. Weight bias: a call to action. J Eat Disord 2016;4(1):1–6.

Eating Disorders in the Primary Care Setting

Amanda Mellowspring, MS, RD/N, CEDS-S

KEYWORDS

- Eating disorders • Anorexia nervosa (AN) • Bulimia nervosa (BN)
- Binge eating disorder (BED) • Avoidant restrictive food intake disorder (ARFID)
- Other specified feeding or eating disorder (OSFED)

KEY POINTS

- Eating disorders are mental health disorders with high medical and psychiatric mortalities.
- Eating disorder behaviors commonly intersect diagnoses and are not dependent on body weight.
- Eating disorders affect across racial, ethnic, gender, and socioeconomic demographics and occur across ages ranging from pediatric to geriatric.
- Eating disorder treatment requires interprofessional care from a variety of disciplines. Careful consideration should be given to seeking out providers with expertise in working with eating disorders owing to the prevalence of misinformation.
- Eating disorder recovery requires ongoing care with various stages of support.

INTRODUCTION

Eating disorders are mental health disorders with complicating medical, psychiatric, and nutritional comorbidities and are among the most deadly mental illnesses.[1–4] In addition to severe medical complications, approximately 26% of those with eating disorders attempt suicide.[1] Common eating disorder diagnoses include anorexia nervosa (AN), bulimia nervosa (BN), binge eating disorder (BED), avoidant restrictive food intake disorder (ARFID), other specified feeding or eating disorder (OSFED), and unspecified feeding or eating disorder (UFED).[5,6] Eating disorders occur across age, gender, racial, ethnic, and socioeconomic variables.[6,7] Effective assessment, intervention, and collaborative treatment are needed to decrease risk factors and increase opportunity for recovery. Presently only about one-third of those with an eating disorder ever receive treatment.[6] In addition to limited knowledge on the subject among medical providers, proper diagnosis and treatment are complicated by medical biases related to race, gender, sexuality, and weight when considering eating disorders.[7–11]

Monte Nido & Affiliates, 6100 SW 76th Street, Miami, FL 33143, USA
E-mail address: amellowspring@montenidoaffiliates.com

Prim Care Clin Office Pract 50 (2023) 103–117
https://doi.org/10.1016/j.pop.2022.10.012 **primarycare.theclinics.com**

Abbreviations	
AN	Anorexia Nervosa
BN	Bulimia Nervosa
BED	Binge Eating Disorder
ARFID	Avoidant Restrictive Food Intake Disorder
OSFED	Other Specified Feeding or Eating Disorder
UFED	Unspecified Feeding or Eating Disorder

Anorexia Nervosa

AN has the highest mortality of all mental disorders and is the most commonly recognized eating disorder, indicative of restrictive eating behaviors.[12] It is notable that in the American Psychiatric Association (2013) *Diagnostic and Statistical Manual of Mental Disorders* (Fifth Edition), diagnostic criteria related to standardized weight assessment measurements and amenorrhea were removed, as noted in **Box 1**.[5,13,14]

This is vital in the assessment and diagnosis of a large percentage of patients, including girls prior to menarche, boys and men of all ages, and patients whose typical body weight exceeds *normal* by standardized body mass index measurements. Men and boys represent 25% of individuals with AN and are at higher risk of death, in part because men and boys are often diagnosed later owing to lack of screening for male subjects and eating disorders.[15]

Bulimia Nervosa

BN is an eating disorder of binge eating and compensatory behaviors, most widely recognized by purging behaviors, such as self-induced vomiting or laxative misuse, as noted in **Box 2**. Although as with other eating disorders BN leads to severe malnutrition, it is less correlated with body weight.[16]

Comorbid mood, anxiety, and substance use disorders are prevalent among patients with BN. More than half of patients with BN have co-occurring anxiety disorders, whereas close to half present with mood disorders.[17] Within racial and ethnic demographics, lifetime prevalence for BN is higher in Latino and African American populations. Athletes of all genders are at higher risk in sports where leanness is the preferred body type or where *cutting weight* is expected.[16,18]

Box 1
Anorexia nervosa diagnostic criteria

A. Restriction of energy intake relative to requirements leading to a significantly low body weight in the context of age, sex, developmental trajectory, and physical health. *Significantly low weight* is defined as a weight that is less than minimally normal or, for children and adolescents, less than that minimally expected.

B. Intense fear of gaining weight or becoming fat, or persistent behavior that interferes with weight gain, even though at a significantly low weight.

C. Disturbance in the way in which one's body weight or shape is experienced, undue influence of body weight or shape on self-evaluation, or persistent lack of recognition of the seriousness of the current low body weight.

Reprinted with permission from the Diagnostic and Statistical Manual of Mental Disorders: DSM-5, 5th ed., pp. 338-339, 345, 350, 334, 353-354 (Copyright © 2013). American Psychiatric Association. All Rights Reserved.

Box 2
Bulimia nervosa diagnostic criteria

A. Recurrent episodes of binge eating. An episode of binge eating is characterized by both of the following:
    a. Eating, in a discrete period of time (eg, within any 2-hour period), an amount of food that is definitely larger than most people would eat during a similar period of time and under similar circumstances.
    b. A sense of lack of control over eating during the episode (eg, a feeling that one cannot stop eating or control what or how much one is eating).

B. Recurrent inappropriate compensatory behavior in order to prevent weight gain, such as self-induced vomiting, misuse of laxatives, diuretics, or other medications, fasting, or excessive exercise.

C. The binge eating and inappropriate compensatory behaviors both occur, on average, at least once a week for 3 months.

D. Self-evaluation is unduly influenced by body shape and weight.

E. The disturbance does not occur exclusively during episodes of anorexia nervosa.

Reprinted with permission from the Diagnostic and Statistical Manual of Mental Disorders: DSM-5, 5th ed., pp. 338-339, 345, 350, 334, 353-354 (Copyright © 2013). American Psychiatric Association. All Rights Reserved.

Binge Eating Disorder

BED is the most common eating disorder among adults in the United States, exceeding 3 times the cases of AN and BN combined.[6] Despite the prevalence of BED, it was only first acknowledged as an independent mental health diagnosis with defining diagnostic criteria that in the American Psychiatric Association (2013) *Diagnostic and Statistical Manual of Mental Disorders* (Fifth Edition), as shown in **Box 3**.[5]

Box 3
Binge eating disorder diagnostic criteria

A. Recurrent episodes of binge eating. An episode of binge eating is characterized by both of the following:
    a. Eating, in a discrete period of time (eg, within any 2-hour period), an amount of food that is definitely larger than what most people would eat in a similar period of time under similar circumstances.
    b. A sense of lack of control over eating during the episode (eg, a feeling that one cannot stop eating or control what or how much one is eating).

B. The binge eating episodes are associated with three (or more) of the following:
    a. Eating much more rapidly than normal.
    b. Eating until feeling uncomfortably full.
    c. Eating large amounts of food when not feeling physically hungry.
    d. Eating alone because of feeling embarrassed by how much one is eating.
    e. Feeling disgusted with oneself, depressed, or very guilty afterward.

C. Marked distress regarding binge eating is present.

D. The binge eating occurs, on average, at least once a week for 3 months.

E. The binge eating is not associated with the recurrent use of inappropriate compensatory behaviors (eg, purging) as in bulimia nervosa and does not occur exclusively during the course of bulimia nervosa or anorexia nervosa.

Reprinted with permission from the Diagnostic and Statistical Manual of Mental Disorders: DSM-5, 5th ed., pp. 338-339, 345, 350, 334, 353-354 (Copyright © 2013). American Psychiatric Association. All Rights Reserved.

Approximately 40% of patients diagnosed with BED are male patients, making BED the most common eating disorder among boys and men and denotes the need for greater awareness of gender biased assessment in eating disorder assessment.[10,11]

Studies estimate as low as 3% of individuals who meet criteria for BED are ever assessed, with estimates between 28% and 45% for those who receive treatment.[7,10]

Avoidant Restrictive Food Intake Disorder

ARFID was delineated as an independent eating disorder with specific diagnostic criteria in the American Psychiatric Association (2013) *Diagnostic and Statistical Manual of Mental Disorders* (Fifth Edition), as shown in **Box 4**. ARFID was previously categorized under *Feeding and Eating Disorders of Infancy or Early Childhood*.[5,13,14] Although selective eating is developmentally typical for young children, the development of ARFID as a mental health diagnosis denotes the more extreme nature of the behavior patterns among all age groups.[19,20] Nearly half of children with ARFID report fear of vomiting or choking, and one-fifth attribute food avoidance to sensory issues.[21]

Other Specified Feeding or Eating Disorder

OSFED is categorized by symptoms of a feeding or eating disorder that causes clinical distress or impairment in social, occupational, or other important areas of functioning, however does not meet the full criteria for any of the disorders in the feeding and eating disorders diagnostic class. A diagnosis might then be assigned that addresses the specific reason the presentation does not meet the specifics of another disorder (eg, BN–low frequency). Examples of OSFED are noted in **Table 1**.[5]

Updates in the American Psychiatric Association (2013) *Diagnostic and Statistical Manual of Mental Disorders* (Fifth Edition) broadened definitions of AN, BN, and

---

Box 4
Avoidant restrictive food intake disorder diagnostic criteria

A. An eating or feeding disturbance (eg, apparent lack of interest in eating or food; avoidance based on the sensory characteristics of food; concern about aversive consequences of eating) as manifested by persistent failure to meet appropriate nutritional and/or energy needs associated with one (or more) of the following:
  a. Significant weight loss (or failure to achieve expected weight gain or faltering growth in children).
  b. Significant nutritional deficiency.
  c. Dependence on enteral feeding or oral nutritional supplements.
  d. Marked interference with psychosocial functioning.

B. The disturbance is not better explained by lack of available food or by an associated culturally sanctioned practice.

C. The eating disturbance does not occur exclusively during the course of anorexia nervosa or bulimia nervosa, and there is no evidence of a disturbance in the way in which one's body weight or shape is experienced.

D. The eating disturbance is not attributable to a concurrent medical condition or not better explained by another mental disorder. When the eating disturbance occurs in the context of another condition or disorder, the severity of the eating disturbance exceeds that routinely associated with the condition or disorder and warrants additional clinical attention.

Reprinted with permission from the Diagnostic and Statistical Manual of Mental Disorders: DSM-5, 5th ed., pp. 338-339, 345, 350, 334, 353-354 (Copyright © 2013). American Psychiatric Association. All Rights Reserved.

Table 1 Examples of other specified feeding or eating disorder	
Example	**Description**
Atypical anorexia nervosa	All of the criteria for anorexia nervosa are met, except that despite significant weight loss, the individual's weight is within or above the normal range.
Bulimia nervosa (of low frequency and/or limited duration)	All of the criteria for bulimia nervosa are met, except that the binge eating and inappropriate compensatory behavior occurs, on average, less than once a week and/or for less than 3 months.
Binge eating disorder (of low frequency and/ or limited duration):	All of the criteria for binge eating disorder are met, except that the binge eating occurs on average less than once a week and/or for less than 3 months.
Purging disorder	Recurrent purging behavior to influence weight or shape (eg, self-induced vomiting, misuse of laxatives, diuretics, or other medications) in the absence of binge eating.
Night eating syndrome	Recurrent episodes of night eating, as manifested by eating after awakening from sleep or by excessive food consumption after the evening meal. There is awareness and recall of the eating. The night eating is not better explained by external influences, such as changes in the individual's sleep-wake cycle or by local social norms. The night eating causes significant distress and/or impairment in functioning. The disordered pattern of eating is not better explained by binge eating disorder or another mental disorder, including substance use, and is not attributable to another medical disorder or to an effect of medication.

Reprinted with permission from the Diagnostic and Statistical Manual of Mental Disorders: DSM-5, 5th ed., pp. 338-339, 345, 350, 334, 353-354 (Copyright © 2013). American Psychiatric Association. All Rights Reserved.

defined BED to more accurately diagnose these eating disorders, although OSFED remains a common diagnosis.[13,14]

Unspecified Feeding or Eating Disorder

UFED applies to presentations in which symptoms characteristic of a feeding and eating disorder that cause clinically significant distress or impairment in social, occupational, or other important areas of functions predominate but do not meet the full criteria for any of the disorders in the feeding and eating disorders diagnostic class.

The UFED category is used in situations in which the clinician chooses not to specify the reason that the criteria are not met for a specific feeding and eating disorder and includes presentation in which there is insufficient information to make a more specific diagnosis (eg, in emergency room settings).[5]

DISCUSSION

Eating disorders are not choices and have multiple biological and psychosocial risk factors, including genetic and environmental factors.[22] Risk factors include personality traits, such as perfectionism and impulsivity, as well as binge eating and dieting behaviors.[23] Early intervention is a key indicator in the success of eating disorder treatment.[24,25]

Assessment

Thorough and informed assessment of patients with an eating disorder should focus on maladaptive behaviors and patterns. Many individuals with eating disorders appear healthy, yet may be extremely ill.[26] The body can temporarily adapt to the stressors of an eating disorder, causing laboratory tests to appear normal, requiring thorough and consistent medical understanding and management.[3,4,24] Subclinical restrictive eating, bingeing, and purging behaviors should not be minimized. Assessment through the combination of interview, physical examination, and laboratory values will provide the most thorough medical assessment, as shown in **Boxes 5** and **6** and **Table 2**.[3,4,27]

Weight bias within health care can interfere with proper diagnosis and treatment. Excessive value placed on weight loss as well as conflation of weight and health regarding all eating disorder diagnoses by providers can delay diagnosis and impede treatment.[3,24] Patients in larger bodies are half as likely as those at a *normal weight* or *underweight* to be diagnosed with an eating disorder.[7]

Medical Complications

Eating disorders create a complex medical and psychological picture with involvement of all organ systems in the body. Although the body can be resilient in managing the stress of eating disorder behaviors, stability can be tenuous and result in serious medical consequences, including death.[24,25]

Through self-starvation indicative of AN and the food avoidance of ARFID, the body will work to compensate for lack of nutrition by conserving energy, resulting in many of the complications depicted in **Table 3**. Laboratory values may falsely appear normal as a result.[24]

The cyclical binge/purge behaviors indicative of BN lead to life-threatening fluctuations in electrolytes and gastrointestinal symptoms. Electrolyte fluctuations can lead to cardiac collapse secondary to the weakened heart muscle.[4]

Box 5
Clinical assessment, interview topics

Body image distress

Fear of weight gain

Restrictive eating

Vomiting

Binge eating

Laxative use

Exercise (excessive, compensatory, or avoidance)

Selective eating

Weight history & weight changes

Gastrointestinal distress

Depression

Anxiety

Substance use

Neurologic examination

Box 6
Clinical assessment, physical examination

Height & weight

Pulse & blood pressure

Dentition

Signs of dehydration

Oral lesions

Esophageal irritation

Skin examination
• Russell signs
• Dry skin
• Cold, mottled extremities

Hair loss or texture changes

Abdominal examination

Extremity examination (edema & cyanosis)

Musculoskeletal examination (weakness)

Cardiac examination

Although the persistent binge behavior associated with BED can lead to weight gain, medical complications resulting from binge behavior are most correlated with health risk factors associated with weight cycling.[3,10,11,28,29] Patients who struggle with BED tend to be of normal or higher-than-average weight, although BED can be diagnosed at any weight.[30]

OSFED and UFED present with variations of the eating disordered behaviors noted in AN, BN, BED, and ARFID and will follow the associated symptoms and thus medical complications, as shown in **Table 3**.[3,4,27] **Fig. 1** provides a visual of the full body involvement.

Table 2
Laboratory results often seen with eating disorders

Anorexia Nervosa	Bulimia Nervosa
High cholesterol	High amylase
Low blood glucose	Low sodium
Elevated liver enzymes	Low potassium
Bradycardia (heart rate <60 beats/min)	Low magnesium
Low white blood cell count (leukopenia)	Metabolic alkalosis
Low red blood cell count (anemia)	Non-gap metabolic acidosis
Low luteinizing hormone, follicle-stimulating hormone, estradiol, or testosterone levels	
Low thyroxine levels (T4)	
Low phosphorus	
Low sodium	
Osteopenia/osteoporosis	

Table 3
Medical complications of eating disorders

AN	BN	BED	General
*	*		Muscle weakness
*	*	*	Difficulty concentrating
AN	**BN**	**BED**	**Gastrointestinal**
	*	*	Gastroesophageal reflux
*			Gastroparesis
*	*	*	Constipation/diarrhea/nausea
	*		Hematemesis
	*		Hematochezia
	*		Tears and/or lesions of the esophagus
	*		Barrett esophagus
*			Early satiety
*			Delayed gastric emptying
*	*	*	Gallbladder involvement
*			Superior mesenteric artery syndrome
AN	**BN**	**BED**	**Cardiovascular**
*	*		Weakened cardiac muscle
*	*		Bradycardia
*	*		Tachycardia
*	*		EKG abnormalities
*	*		Cardiovascular collapse secondary to refeeding syndrome
*	*		Dizziness, fainting/syncope
*			Anemia
*			Low blood cell count
	*		Low potassium
*		*	Poor circulation
*	*	*	Edema
AN	**BN**	**BED**	**Endocrine/Gynecologic**
*	*		Low hormones (aldosterone, estrogen, testosterone)
*	*		Thyroid hormone disruption
*			Low blood glucose secondary to depleted liver glycogen stores
*			High cholesterol (resolves with refeeding)
*	*		Bone loss/osteopenia/osteoporosis
*	*		Amenorrhea
*	*		Thinning of hair/brittle nails
*	*		Dry skin
*			Fine hair on body (lanugo)
*			Poor wound healing
*	*		Impaired immune functioning
AN	**BN**	**BED**	**Oral/Dental**
	*		Erosion of enamel/tooth decay
*	*		Lesions in the mouth
	*		Parotid hypertrophy

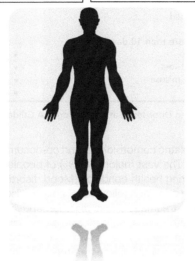

Brain Anxiety, Depression	**Mouth** Tooth decay, jaw pain, swollen parotid glands

Heart Irregular heartbeat, BP, chol, cardiac failure, poor circulation	**Throat/Esophagus** Reflux, irritation, lesions/tears, Barretts esophagus
Endocrine Low hormones, thyroid abnormalities, amenorrhea, low BG	**Gastrointestinal** Diarrhea, bloating, delayed gastric emptying, gallbladder, kidney
Bone Bone loss, low bone density, osteopenia	**Skin** Dry skin, brittle nails, lanugo, hair loss, Russells signs

Fig. 1. Medical complications of eating disorders. BG, blood glucose; BP, blood pressure; chol, cholesterol.

Refeeding Syndrome

Nutritional rehabilitation is vital to the treatment of all eating disorder diagnoses. Without regard to body weight, it should be validated that any patient presenting with eating disordered behaviors is poorly nourished and requires nutritional rehabilitation for medical stabilization.[3,24]

Most treatment interventions require noncompulsory feeding by mouth with some programs offering voluntary enteral feeding when indicated. Total parenteral nutrition can also be used in hospital settings to nourish patients while resolving gastrointestinal complications or obstruction.[3,4] Involuntary enteral or parenteral feeding is controversial and rarely used even in extreme cases.[31,32]

Refeeding syndrome is a critical medical complication of nutritional rehabilitation with the potential for lethal cardiovascular collapse.[3,4,24] The 2 factors associated with refeeding syndrome are reduced cardiovascular mass secondary to weight loss and electrolyte abnormalities secondary to malnutrition and behavior engagement.[4] Risk factors and symptoms of refeeding syndrome are shown in **Table 4**.

INTERVENTIONS

In addition to medical complications, there are additional psychosocial factors that can complicate treatment interventions for patients with an eating disorder. Among adolescents with an eating disorder, fewer than 1 in 5 have received treatment, although ranked as the third leading chronic disease among adolescents.[2,33] Empirical evidence suggests that, despite profound impairment, only 26% of those with eating disorders receive any consultation for symptoms, and fewer still engage in empirically supported treatments.[22,34]

Table 4
Refeeding syndrome

Patient Risk Factors	Signs of Refeeding Syndrome

• Severely malnourished
• Chronically undernourished
• Acutely undernourished
  (little or no intake for more than 10 days)
• Significant alcohol intake
• Postbariatric with weight loss
• Diuretic, laxative, insulin misuse
	• Electrolyte abnormalities
	  ○ Low phosphorus
	  ○ Low potassium
	  ○ Low magnesium
	• Edema
	• Muscle weakness
	• Cognitive delay
	• Gastrointestinal disruption

Data from Academy for Eating Disorders. Eating Disorders: A Guide to Medical Care. AED Report 2021, 4th ed.

Suicidal ideation, psychiatric comorbidities, and co-occurring substance use disorder are complicating factors. The vast majority (97%) of people hospitalized for an eating disorder have a co-occurring health condition. Mood disorders, like major depression, are the primary underlying condition followed by anxiety disorders, such as obsessive-compulsive disorder, post-traumatic stress disorder, and substance use disorder.[35]

Weight bias within health care can interfere with proper diagnosis and treatment. Excessive value placed on weight loss as well as conflation of weight and health by providers can delay diagnosis and impede treatment.[24] Although less than 6% of people with eating disorders are medically diagnosed as *underweight*, people in larger bodies are half as likely as those at a *normal weight* or *underweight* to be diagnosed with an eating disorder.[6,7]

Lack of insight regarding the severity of illness and ambivalence related to behavior change are common complicating factors and should be considered in determining treatment approach and interventions for many patients with eating disorders.[3,24] Access to care, including knowledgeable providers, financial means, and physical location, must also be considered when determining treatment.[13,35]

Interprofessional Care Team

The treatment of eating disorders requires interdisciplinary collaboration of the professionals on the care team both among themselves and in coordination with the patient.[24,25,36] The family and/or social support system of a patient also plays an integral role in the treatment and progress in recovery.[26,37–39] Although many medical diseases are diagnosed, assessed, and managed by a medical provider, in eating disorder treatment, all providers must be able to engage directly with the patient to effect long-term, sustainable behavior change. **Table 5** lists the core members of an

Table 5
Interprofessional care team

Team Members	Role(s) in Treatment
Mental health provider(s)	Support patients in exploring behavior change, interpersonal effectiveness, family/social dynamics, self-efficacy, trauma processing
Dietitian	Support patients with behavior change through dietary recommendations and nutritional guidance
Medical provider(s)	Medical oversight and monitoring
Psychiatrist	Psychiatric medication management

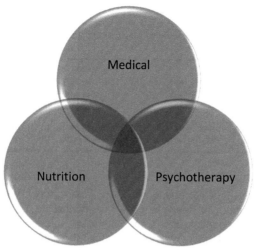

Fig. 2. Collaboration of treatment care team.

interprofessional eating disorder care team and their general roles in treatment. **Fig. 2** depicts the vital overlap and engagement of the core treatment components: medical, psychotherapy, and nutrition. The interprofessional dynamic of these modalities is vital to the behavior change necessary to result in long-term recovery.[24,36,40–42]

Levels of Care

The complicating interplay of medical, psychological, and nutritional needs for eating disorder treatment requires a high degree of expertise to assess, monitor, and support

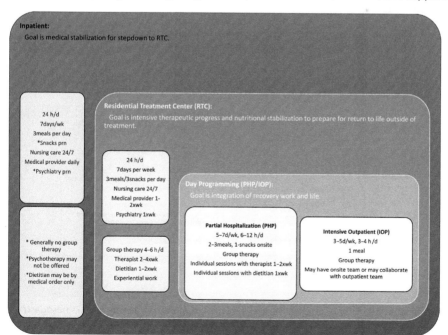

Fig. 3. Levels of treatment. prn, as needed. *Inpatient eating disorder–focused programs offer these services as a standard of care. Standard inpatient hospital settings do not.

Box 7
Criteria considered in determining level of care needed for eating disorder treatment

Medical Status	Structure Needed for Eating/Gaining Weight
Suicidality	Ability to control compulsive exercising
Weight as percentage of healthy body weight	Purging behavior (laxatives and diuretics)
Motivation to recover	Environmental stress
Cooccurring disorders	Geographic availability

Data from American Psychiatric Association. Practice guideline for the treatment of patients with eating disorders, 3rd ed. American Psychiatric Association; 2006.

patients in long-term behavior change once medically stable. Various levels of care exist along a continuum of need: inpatient, residential treatment center, and day programming–partial hospitalization, and intensive outpatient levels of care are commonly accepted as higher levels of care within the eating disorder care process. In considering levels of care treatment for eating disorders, the primary differentiators are hours of treatment, level of medical oversight, nutritional intervention, and therapeutic engagement, as shown in **Fig. 3**.[24,25,37]

Box 7 depicts criteria put forth by the *American Psychiatric Association Practice Guidelines* considered in determining the appropriate level of care. **Fig. 4** uses the levels of care to depict the medical criteria within this level of care as shown in the *American Psychiatric Association Practice Guidelines*.[25]

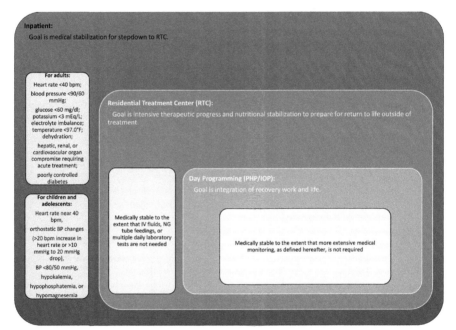

Fig. 4. Medical criteria in determining level of care. IV, intravenous; NG, nasogastric.[43] (*Adapted from* La Via M, Kaye WH, et al. Anorexia nervosa: criteria for levels of care. Paper presented at the annual meeting of the Eating Disorders Research Society, Cambridge, Mass, November 5–7, 1998.)

SUMMARY

Eating disorders are life-threatening mental health disorders that can involve all organ systems in the body and are associated with complicating psychosocial factors requiring collaborative care. The complex medical, psychological, and nutritional aspects of eating disorders create the need for an intricate care team and interprofessional treatment approach.

Informed assessment and early intervention are vital to increase efficacy of treatment and long-term recovery. Misinformation and medical bias regarding weight, gender, and race adversely affect assessment and treatment measures. Interprofessional care, including medical monitoring, nutritional rehabilitation, and mental health counseling, including health-related behavior change addressed by medical providers, dietitians, psychiatrists, and mental health providers, is the benchmark to support enduring recovery for those suffering from eating disorders.

CLINICS CARE POINTS

- Patients of all body sizes can have life-threatening eating disorders.
- The majority of patients with eating disorders are not visibly emaciated.
- Eating disorders require a multidisciplinary team approach, including but not limited to knowledgeable medical, psychological, and nutritional care providers.

DISCLOSURE

The author has nothing to disclose.

REFERENCES

1. Arcelus J, Mitchell AJ, Wales J, et al. Mortality rates in patients with anorexia nervosa and other eating disorders. A meta-analysis of 36 studies. Arch Gen Psychiatry 2011;68(7):724–31.
2. Birmingham C, Beumont P. Medical management of eating disorders: a practical handbook for health care professionals. Cambridge, UK: Cambridge University Press; 2004.
3. Gaudiani J. Sick enough: a guide to the medical complications of eating disorders. Routledge; 2019.
4. Mehler P, Andersen A. Eating disorders: a guide to medical care and complications. 3rd ed. Baltimore: Johns Hopkins University Press; 2017.
5. American Psychiatric Association. Diagnostic and statistical manual of mental disorders. 5th ed. Arlington, VA: American Psychiatric Association; 2013.
6. Hudson J, Hiripi E, Pope Jr HG, et al. The prevalence and correlates of eating disorders in the National Comorbidity Survey Replication. Bio Psych 2007; 61(3):348–58.
7. Nagata J, Garber A, Tabler JL, et al. Prevalence and Correlates of Disordered Eating Behaviors Among Young adults with Overweight or Obesity. J Gen Intern Med 2018;33(8):1337–43.
8. Becker A, Franko D, Speck A, et al. Ethnicity and differential access to care for eating disorder symptoms. Int J Eat Disord 2003;33(2):205–12.
9. Deloitte Access Economics. The Social and Economic Cost of Eating Disorders in the United States of America: A Report for the Strategic Training Initiative for the Prevention of Eating Disorders and the Academy for Eating Disorders. 2020.

https://www.hsph.harvard.edu/striped/report-economic-costs-of-eating-disorders/. [Accessed 28 March 2022].

10. Westerberg D, Waitz M. Binge-eating disorder. Osteopathic Fam Physician 2013; 5(6):230–3.

11. Bacon Lindo. Health at every size: the surprising truth about your weight. Dallas, TX: BenBella Books, Inc.; 2010.

12. Smink F, van Hoeken D, Hoek H. Epidemiology of Eating Disorders: Incidence, Prevalence and Mortality Rates. Curr Psychiatry Rep 2012;14:406–14.

13. Call C, Walsh B, Attia E. From DSM-IV to DSM-5: changes to eating disorder diagnoses. Curr Opin Psychiatry 2013;26(6):532–6.

14. American Psychiatric Association. Diagnostic and statistical manual of mental disorders, text revision. 4th. Arlington: American Psychiatric Publishing; 2000.

15. Mond J, Mitchison D, Hay P. Prevalence and implications of eating disordered behavior in men. In: Cohn L, Lemberg R, editors. Current findings on males with eating disorders. Philadelphia, PA: Routledge; 2014. p. 15–7.

16. Rushing J, Jones L, Carney C. Bulimia Nervosa: A Primary Care Review. Prim Care Companion J Clin Psychiatry 2003;5(5):217–24.

17. Ulfvebrand S, Birgegard A, Norring C, et al. Psychiatric comorbidity in women and men with eating disorders results from a large clinical database. Psych Res 2015;230(2):294–9.

18. Marques L, Alegria M, Becker AE, et al. Comparative Prevalence, Correlates of Impairment, and Service Utilization for Eating Disorders across U.S. Ethnic Groups: Implications for Reducing Ethnic Disparities in Health Care Access for Eating Disorders. Int J Eat Disord 2011;44(5):412–20.

19. Bryant-Waugh R, Micali N, Cooke L, et al. Development of the Pica, ARFID, and Rumination Disorder Interview, a multi-informant, semi-structured interview of feeding disorders across the lifespan: A pilot study for ages 10–22. Int J Eat Disord 2019;52(4):378–87.

20. Todisco P. Avoidant/Restrictive Food Intake Disorder (ARFID) in Adults. In: Manzato E, Cuzzalaro M, Donini LM, editors. Hidden and lesser-known disordered eating behaviors in medical and psychiatric conditions. Cham: Springer; 2022. p. 103–21.

21. Nicely T, Lane-Loney S, Masciulli E, et al. Prevalence and characteristics of avoidant/restrictive food intake disorder in a cohort of young patients in day treatment for eating disorders. J Eat Disord 2014;2(1):1.

22. Jacobi C, Hayward C, de Zwaan M, et al. Coming to terms with risk factors for eating disorders: application of risk terminology and suggestions for a general taxonomy. Psychopharmacol Bull 2004;130:19–65.

23. Hilbert A, Pike K, Goldschmidt AB, et al. Risk factors across the eating disorders. Psych Res 2014;220(1–2):500–6.

24. Academy for Eating Disorders. Eating disorders: a guide to medical care. 4th ed. Reston, VA: AED Report; 2021.

25. American Psychiatric Association. Practice guideline for the treatment of patients with eating disorders. 3rd ed. Washington, DC: American Psychiatric Association; 2006.

26. Bulik C, Blake L, Austin J, et al. Genetics of eating disorders: What the clinician needs to know. Psych Clin 2019;42(1):59–73.

27. Setnick J. The eating disorders clinical pocket guide: quick reference for healthcare providers. Dallas, TX: Snack Time Press; 2005.

28. Lahti-Koski M, Mannisto S, Pietinen P, et al. Prevalence of weight cycling and its relation to health indicators in Finland. Obes Res 2005;13(2):333–41.

29. Kakainami L, Knauper B, Brunet J. Weight cycling is associated with adverse cardiometabolic markers in a cross-sectional representative US sample. J Epidemial Community Health 2020;74:662–7.

30. Heal D, Gosden J. What pharmacological interventions are effective in binge-eating disorder? Insights from a critical evaluation of the evidence from clinical trials. Int J Obes 2022;46:677–95.

31. Hale M, Logomarsino J. The use of enteral nutrition in the treatment of eating disorders: a systematic review. Eating and Weight Disorders-Studies on Anorexia. Bulimia Obes 2019;24(2):179–98.

32. Hindley K, Fenton C, McIntosh J. A systematic review of enteral feeding by nasogastric tube in young people with eating disorders. J Eat Disord 2021;9:90.

33. Swanson S, Crow S, Le Grange D, et al. Prevalence and Correlates of Eating Disorders in Adolescents: Results From the National Comorbidity Survey Replication Adolescent Supplement. Arch Gen Psychiatry 2011;68(7):714–23.

34. Wittchen H, Jacobi F. Size and burden of mental disorders in Europe — A critical review and appraisal of 27 studies. Eur Neuropsychopharmacol 2005;15(4): 357–76.

35. Murray S. Updates in the treatment of eating disorders in 2018: a year in review in eating disorders: The Journal of Treatment & Prevention. Eat Disord 2019; 27(1):6–17.

36. Tholking M, Mellowspring A, Girard-Eberle S, et al. American Dietetic Association: Standards of Practice and Standards of Professional Performance for Registered Dietitians (Competent, Proficient, and Expert) in Disordered Eating and Eating Disorders (DE and ED). J Am Diet Assoc 2011;111(8).

37. Anderson L, Reilly E, Berner L, et al. Treating Eating Disorders at Higher Levels of Care: Overview and Challenges. Curr Psychiatry Rep 2017;19:48.

38. LeGrange D, Lock J, Loeb K, et al. Academy for eating disorders position paper: The role of the family in eating disorders. Int J Eat Disord 2010;43(1):1–5.

39. Murray SB, Anderson LK, Roxanne. Adapting family-based treatment for adolescent anorexia nervosa across higher levels of patient care. Innovations in Family Therapy for Eating Disorders. New York: Routledge; 2016. p. 29–40.

40. Jansen A, Broekmate J, Heymans M. Cue-exposure vs self-control in the treatment of binge eating: A pilot study. Behav Res Ther 1992;30(3):235–41.

41. Schebendach J, Mayer L, Devlin MJ, et al. Dietary energy density and diet variety as risk factors for relapse in anorexia nervosa: A replication. Int J Eat Disord 2012; 45(1):79–84.

42. Steinglass J, Albano A, Simpson HB, et al. Confronting fear using exposure and response prevention for anorexia nervosa: a randomized controlled pilot study. Int J Eat Disord 2014;47(2):174–80.

43. La Via M. 3.1 Screening, Diagnosis, and Comorbidity of Eating Disorders. J Am Acad Child Adolesc Psychiatry 2016;55(10):S88.

Obsessive Compulsive Disorders in the Primary Care Setting

Robin Newburn, DO

KEYWORDS

- OCD • Primary care • Mental health

KEY POINTS

- Obsessive-compulsive disorder (OCD) historical background: a brief discussion highlighting the historical development of OCD as a diagnosis and clinical entity, and the ways in which it was considered by the medical and scientific communities and provided the foundation for current concepts.
- *OCD diagnosis*: a discussion about the clinical features of OCD, the diagnostic criteria that must be met, and the tools currently used to confirm the diagnosis.
- *OCD treatment:* an examination of the current standard of care and best practices related to the treatment options available to a primary care provider (PCP) for OCD in its various forms.
- *OCD case study:* a fictitious case that could possibly be encountered in the primary care setting is used to demonstrate the importance of appropriate diagnosis, treatment, and clinical judgment in a complex OCD patient.

Nothing in life is to be feared; it is only to be understood. Now is the time to understand more so that we may fear less.

—Marie Curie

Sometimes in pop culture, we see the term OCD used loosely and often trivialized in a ridiculing manner when in fact, it is no laughing matter, and many are suffering. As medical professionals, we have a responsibility to destigmatize and educate our communities about this condition and mental health in general.

This article will discuss OCD and its diagnosis and treatment from a primary care perspective.

It will discuss the history, evolution, and impact of this condition, and the ways in which it is diagnosed and treated, and then conclude by presenting a clinical case study for consideration.

Ohio University Heritage College of Osteopathic Medicine, 6785 Bobcat Way, Dublin, OH 43016, USA
E-mail address: newburnr@ohio.edu

Prim Care Clin Office Pract 50 (2023) 119–125
https://doi.org/10.1016/j.pop.2022.10.001
0095-4543/23/© 2022 Elsevier Inc. All rights reserved.

Obsessive-compulsive disorder (OCD) is a condition that is commonly encountered in primary care practices across the nation every day—sometimes even unbeknownst to the physicians and other providers who care for the whole health of patients while having the opportunity to get to know them quite well. This certainly reinforces the importance of taking the time to perform a thorough history and physical to uncover the issues that a patient may not be very willing to divulge voluntarily. Ultimately, this knowledge will benefit the patient by ensuring that they receive the best care and treatment for a condition that can be very disruptive and even debilitating for some.

According to the National Institute of Mental Health, approximately 1% of the United States population is affected by OCD, with about one-third of all cases presenting during childhood,[1] and the worldwide prevalence is approximately 2% of the general population.[2]

It is estimated that of the 1% of people who are diagnosed with OCD, approximately 50% of them have serious impairment, 35% are moderately impaired, and 15% have mild symptoms.[1]

In many cities and communities across the United States, a common concern that is often voiced by primary care providers is that there seems to be a shortage of mental health services, making it difficult to find psychiatrists and clinical psychologists to refer patients to for the diagnosis and initiation of treatment. For this reason, primary care providers should be familiar and comfortable with diagnostic criteria and treatment options for commonly encountered conditions such as OCD.

The Diagnostic and Statistical Manual (DSM)-V has well-defined diagnostic criteria for OCD, which have been revised in recent years, and are outlined as follows:[3]

1. The presence of obsessions or compulsions or both,
2. Obsessions are recurrent and persistent thoughts, urges, or images that are intrusive and cause distress or anxiety,
3. Compulsions are repetitive behaviors or mental acts that a person feels compelled to perform to relieve the anxiety that the obsessions are causing,
4. The person attempts to suppress, ignore, or neutralize the obsessions or compulsions with some other thought or action,
5. The obsessions and/or compulsions take up more than 1 hour per day, or cause clinically significant distress or social, occupational, or other impairment,
6. The disturbance is not attributable to the physiologic effects of a substance or another medical condition, and
7. The disturbance cannot be better explained by the presence of another mental disorder.

The exact cause of OCD is unknown; however, some risk factors have been both theorized and identified such as having a first degree relative with the condition; an anatomic predisposition due to the presence of abnormalities in certain areas of the brain such as the cerebral cortex and basal ganglia, childhood trauma, and very rarely, OCD may develop as a sequela of pediatric autoimmune neuropsychiatric disorder associated with streptococcal infections.[1]

Regarding brain anatomy, some imaging studies have shown strong evidence of increased activity in brain regions that form a cortico-striato-thalamo-cortical loop, which is the reason deep brain stimulation may be a viable and beneficial treatment option in some cases.[1]

Recommended treatment of OCD typically consists of medication and/or psychotherapy such as cognitive behavioral therapy (CBT) and a specific type of CBT called exposure response prevention (ERP). With ERP, the patient is coached through refraining from engaging in compulsions during repeated exposures to a provocative stimulus or situation.[4]

For example, a patient with a hand-washing compulsion following touching certain objects, may be asked to touch a perceived or imagined unclean surface, and is then ethically and professionally coached and guided through the distress of not being permitted to wash their hands afterward. Cognitive behavior therapy relies on techniques that are centered around recognizing and reframing thought patterns to align with reality.[4]

For example, a child with a checking compulsion has insomnia because they are spending the night checking under the bed for a monster instead of sleeping. With CBT, they can be rationally reassured that the concept of a monster actually residing under the bed planning to do them harm has no tangible or logical evidence that is reality-based.

Another form of nonpharmacological treatment is transcranial magnetic stimulation (TMS), which is reserved for cases that are refractory to other forms of treatment. TMS is noninvasive procedure in which an electromagnetic coil is placed on the forehead.

This procedure is thought to work by stimulating neurons located in brain regions showing decreased activity in depression.[5] It has long been known that dysregulation of the striatal serotonergic system is a primary pathologic condition in OCD,[5] and therefore, pharmacologic treatment with the selective serotonin reuptake inhibitor (SSRI) class remains the gold standard for symptom management in OCD. Although the exact mechanism of action is not definitively known, past studies have shown a high degree of symptom relief when compared with other antidepressant classes.[6] SSRIs with proven efficacy and FDA approval for OCD are fluoxetine, fluvoxamine, paroxetine, and sertraline.[5]

In some cases, the addition of an antipsychotic agent may be both necessary and beneficial for the patient, especially in the presence of a tic disorder. Some studies have shown evidence of dysfunction or dysregulation of the glutamatergic system in people suffering from OCD, which has led to the testing of glutamate modulating agents as a potential treatment option.[7] It is often said that there is nothing new under the sun, and when it comes to most human afflictions of the body, mind, and spirit, this is surely the case. Certainly, mental illness has existed since the beginning of human history. It is well known that humans have a dark and storied past encompassing centuries of misunderstanding and maltreatment of people with mental health disorders. Documented history tells us that many people were locked away in institutions and asylums and endured the most appalling conditions and the most inhumane experiments—many unknowingly sacrificing their lives for scientific advancement. Documentation and description of OCD has been discovered as early as 1621, by Robert Burton in his book "The Anatomy of Melancholy".[8] Phillipe Pinel (1745–1826) helped revolutionize the way that institutions and asylums were treating patients, moving from forcible restraints to promoting a gentle, supportive, and cheerful atmosphere that involved the family and friends of the patient.[9]

The building blocks of the foundation of our modern understanding of OCD were developed in the nineteenth century, during which time the term neurosis was coined which described the disorder as a neuropathological condition not caused by an anatomic abnormality.[8]

Scientific experts of that era offered treatment modalities such as psychology, mesmerism, and phrenology for a disorder whose origin they could actually neither discern nor agree on. Some thought the cause was emotional, whereas others maintained that it was either intellectual or due to a disorder of the human will.[8]

According to Sigmund Freud (1856–1930), who is considered by many to be the father of modern era psychology, what is happening in someone with OCD, is that the mind responds maladaptively to conflicts between unacceptable, unconscious sexual or aggressive impulses and the demands of conscience and reality.[8]

There are common themes to be aware of that may be categorized under the more general term OCD[10]:

1. Fear of contamination (germaphobia),
2. Fear of harm (unlocked doors, open windows),
3. Excessive concern with order, symmetry, and neatness (spices alphabetized with labels arranged by color),
4. Obsessions with the physical body and/or bodily functions (breathing, defecating), and
5. Undesirable or intrusive thoughts (harming someone, going to hell).

Hoarding has gained a great deal of attention in the past several years, with the sensationalistic approach often characteristic of TV show interviews. These interviews feature conversations with people who have been rescued from their hoard, along with their very concerned loved ones.

With the advent of shows such as "Hoarders" and "Hoarding: Buried Alive!" and the explosion of social media, the public has had an intimate, never-before-seen front row seat view to a way of life previously unknown or unimaginable to the average person. It could be argued that this has helped society recognize that hoarding is a mental health disorder and not a lifestyle choice.

Increased awareness has hopefully encouraged more people to seek help for themselves or their loved ones. It is important to realize that hoarding is a form of OCD, and was once listed as an obsessive-compulsive personality disorder in the DSM-IV.

However, for years, many experts had thought that it deserved to be in a category of its own, owing to the unique set of features that are the hallmarks of this disorder. Therefore, it is now described as a separate entity in the DSM-V as Hoarding Disorder but remains classified under "Obsessive Compulsive and Related Disorders".[10]

Most primary care physicians and other providers will not have an opportunity to visit patients in their homes and are, therefore, unable to bear witness to the full impact Hoarding Disorder can have on patients, their families, and friends. In the office setting, it would be challenging to ascertain whether a patient is suffering from this disorder unless they willingly divulge that information. In the context of the standard history-taking interview, we do not typically inquire about the details of living conditions, and perhaps we should. Agoraphobia is a panic disorder, which can be present in a patient with OCD, in terms of the obsessions and/or compulsions being of a severe enough nature that they prevent the person from being able to function outside of their home environment. In that case, they develop an extreme and pathologic fear of being outside of the home—originating from the Greek root word "agora" meaning "place of assembly" or "open space".[11]

In the 1997 film "As Good As It Gets", directed by James L. Brooks, one of the main characters is a writer named Mr. Udall who is portrayed by Jack Nicholson. He suffers from a severe form of OCD, and although he is able to leave his home, he encounters many distressing challenges along the way, which makes it very difficult and almost impossible for him to engage with people and to form meaningful connections and relationships. As he walks around Manhattan, he very carefully and methodically steps over sidewalk cracks, places a handkerchief over doorknobs before touching them, and brings his own plastic eating utensils to restaurants.

It is often said that art imitates life, and therefore we must be cognizant of challenges such as those experienced by Mr. Udall because they pertain to caring for our patients in the primary care setting. We may accomplish this by being mindful and empathetic with regard to the barriers they may face merely by making an appointment and coming into the office.

We must be able to provide a safe and welcoming environment for all patients to avoid provoking or exacerbating anxiety-related conditions.

It is widely known that billionaire business magnate Howard Hughes (1905–1976) suffered from OCD and that he waged a silent but sometimes public war with his mental health, during an era predating SSRIs. During his lifetime, he was one of the wealthiest people in the world and would have been able to afford the most current, innovative, and state-of-the-art treatment money could buy. Even with all of his resources, he was unable to escape the grip of OCD. Many primary care providers are using self-assessment questionnaires, such as the PHQ-9 as part of a routine physical examination, to help paint a more complete picture of whole health status. There are assessment tools for OCD as well, such as the Yale-Brown Obsessive Compulsive Scale (Y-BOCS), a 10-item scale that includes a symptom checklist and can be administered by the patient or clinician.

Using or creating a similar scale for patients in the office could prove to be a valuable and effective tool for gaging the severity and extent of OCD.

CASE STUDY

Michael Spencer is a 37-year-old single man residing with his 78-year-old mother and 42-year-old brother in a small 3-bedroom home, located on a busy street in a suburban neighborhood. Three years ago Michael and his family were living in a different state but were forced to evacuate emergently due to an extreme natural disaster, which resulted in hundreds of casualties, including 2 people he was very close to— a cousin and a childhood friend. He has never been married, has no children, and has always lived with his mother. His parents divorced when he was in his teens, and he has not had a relationship with his father since then. He graduated cum laude with a B.S. degree in biochemical engineering from an Ivy League university, and quickly secured a job with a research and engineering company where he had worked for 12 years.

He has not been employed in the last 3 years due to the fact that he sleeps all day, and is awake all night flushing the toilet hundreds of times and washing his hands in the sink with the water running continuously. His mother has reported struggling to pay a water bill that has quadrupled in the last few months. Michael has also developed mutism in the last 2 years, and keeps his eyes closed while moving about the home. In the last year, he began refusing to leave the home, and also stopped bathing.

He has never smoked, consumed alcohol, or used any recreational substances.

Before 3 years, he had no history of medical or psychiatric diagnoses, and no history of trauma, abuse, illness, infections, surgeries, or hospitalizations. He takes no medications or supplements and consumes a regular diet consisting of meals that are prepared by his mother. It has only been in the last year that the family decided that Michael needed medical attention. He has been hospitalized, evaluated by 3 psychiatrists, and received a diagnosis of severe OCD with underlying psychosis. SSRIs and atypical antipsychotic medications were all ineffective, and he was not deemed a candidate for CBT due to his nonverbal state. TMS was recommended but his mother, who is now his legal guardian and power of attorney, refused to authorize consent for this treatment. A social worker even recommended that Michael be placed in a long-term care facility. Ultimately, his family thought that the best option was to apply for disability benefits for Michael, and to continue caring for him at home.

He is persuaded by his family to go for a car ride and presents to the primary care office with his mother.

The following vital signs are recorded:

Height: 6 ft 2 in

Weight: 240 lbs.

BP: unable to obtain due to uncooperativeness Pulse: 78.

Temperature: 98.2°F.

O_2 sat: 97%

On general observation, he is slouched in a chair with his eyes closed and not responding when greeted or asked questions. His appearance is generally unkempt, with body odor and disheveled clothing—shirt is wrinkled, inside out, and misbuttoned, and he is wearing shoes without socks.

Discussion questions:

1. Do you agree with Michael's diagnosis?
2. What could have possibly triggered the onset of Michael's condition?
3. Has the delay in seeking treatment affected his current condition?
4. Is it possible for Michael's condition to improve?
5. Is it too late for TMS to be effective, if Michael's mother were to change her mind?
6. Do you agree with the family's decision to keep him at home versus a facility?
7. How can you best support Michael and his family as his PCP?

The case of Michael Spencer is representative of the fact that there are people living with OCD who have comorbid psychiatric diagnoses that add a layer of complexity to successful treatment outcomes. However, it is important to remember that most patients presenting in the primary care setting with OCD symptoms will more than likely fall into the mild or moderate levels of severity and without underlying psychiatric diagnoses. As mentioned previously, primary care clinicians are often the first line of engagement in the diagnosis and treatment of OCD and should be able to have some level of knowledge and expertise in this role.

In summary, some Clinics Care Points for successful interactions, diagnosis, and treatment of patients with OCD are listed below.

CLINICS CARE POINTS

- Avoid a chaotic, rushed environment and instead create a calm, caring, safe, and welcoming clinical space for patient evaluation.
- During the encounter, gather objective data by using an assessment tool such as the Y-BOCS and take care to set aside enough time to administer.
- Review the DSM-V diagnostic criteria with patient and their support person(s) to help destigmatize OCD and help patients understand and accept the diagnosis, reassure them that it is a disorder, not a decision.
- Be comfortable initiating SSRI therapy while also referring to clinical psychologist for counseling and CBT, and be willing to titrate, as a higher dose is typically recommended when treating OCD when compared with depression.[12]

- Maintain close follow-up and check-ins via in-person and telehealth appointments as well as phone calls at least monthly.[12]
- Be willing and available to participate in periodic interdisciplinary care team meetings with mental health counselor and social worker, if applicable.

DISCLOSURE

The author hereby affirms that this is original content, and discloses that they have no personal, professional, or financial conflict of interest with regard to the material presented.

REFERENCES

1. Available at: nimh.org.
2. Available at: https://pubmed.ncbi.nlm.nih.gov.
3. Diagnostic and Statistical Manual of Mental Disorders and OCD(ocduk.org).
4. Hezel D, Simpson HB. Exposure and response prevention for obsessive-compulsive disorder: A review and new directions. Indian J Psychiatry 2019 Jan;61(Suppl 1):S85–92.
5. Available at: mayoclinic.org.
6. pharmacoltoxicol.biomedcentral.com.
7. 'Harmonizing the Neurobiology and Treatment of Obsessive-Compulsive Disorder'– Goodman, Storch, Sheth. Am J Psychiatry 2021;178(1):17–29.
8. Stanford Medicine Obsessive-Compulsive Related Disorders(med.stanford.edu/ocd/treatment/history/html).
9. Medicine An Illustrated History, 1987 edition – Albert S. Lyons, M.D., and R. Joseph Petrocelli, II, M.D., p.511.
10. psychologytoday.com.
11. Available at: https://www.britannica.com.
12. Janardhan YC, Sundar AS, Math SB. Clinical practice guidelines for Obsessive-Compulsive Disorder. Indian J Psychiatry 2017;59(Suppl 1):S74–90.

Postpartum Depression
Screening and Collaborative Management

Tabatha Wells, MD

KEYWORDS

- Postpartum depression • Perinatal mood disorders
- Edinburgh postpartum depression scale

KEY POINTS

- Perinatal mood disorders can have short- and long-term effects for all members of the family.
- Screening for perinatal mood disorders should occur at least once during the postpartum period for all patients and more frequently if risk factors are present.
- Treatment options should include collaborative care models, family-focused interventions, therapy, and pharmacologic management if indicated.

INTRODUCTION

Pregnancy is generally viewed as a happy time in the pregnant person's life marking a new role as a parent.[1] For some, however, pregnancy causes great stress in part because of cultural stigmas, socioeconomic status, and gender discrimination, to name a few.[2] This stress can lead to the onset of perinatal mood disorders.[3] Mental health during the perinatal period (pregnancy and the year postpartum) is a serious worldwide concern because anxiety and depression during this time are leading causes of disability.[4] Women are sensitive to hormones and develop depressive symptoms during menses, pregnancy, postpartum, and menopause but are more likely to develop depression or anxiety during the perinatal period than at any other point in their lives.[5] Suicide is a leading cause of maternal death in the first year after delivery. In fact, it is a more common cause of mortality than postpartum hemorrhage or hypertensive disorders.[5–7] Parental depression, no matter when it occurs, effects the whole family. Perinatal depression and other mood disorders specifically can cause short- and long-term effects for all members of the family.[8]

DEFINITIONS

Perinatal mood disorders are separated into multiple categories: depressive disorders, anxiety disorders, and psychosis. Symptoms during and after pregnancy are caused by stress, metabolic changes, and hormone changes.[5]

PO Box 372, Mahomet, IL 61853, USA
E-mail address: tabathawellsmd@gmail.com

Prim Care Clin Office Pract 50 (2023) 127–142
https://doi.org/10.1016/j.pop.2022.10.011
0095-5543/23/© 2022 Elsevier Inc. All rights reserved.

Postpartum Blues

It is important to distinguish between postpartum blues and postpartum or perinatal depression. Postpartum blues, or commonly referred to as "baby blues," occurs during the first 2 weeks postpartum and is not considered a perinatal mood disorder.[9] It occurs most typically in the first few days after delivery, often with the onset of the change from colostrum to mature milk, and resolves within 2 weeks. Symptoms are unsettling and unpredictable, but do not impair function, or only causes mild dysfunction. Postpartum blues is never accompanied by suicidal ideation. Symptoms include crying with no known cause, excessive worrying, sadness, anxiety, mood swings, sleep disturbance/insomnia, headache, forgetfulness, exhaustion, poor concentration, changes in appetite, negative feelings toward baby, and irritability.[10] Treatment is not needed per se, because all patients need is empathy, reassurance, comfort, encouragement, and emotional support. If symptoms last for more than 2 weeks, patients should be evaluated for a perinatal mood disorder. One theory for the cause of postpartum blues is that the mood changes are caused by abrupt hormone withdrawal of estrogen and progesterone.[11] Evidence of this hypothesis is that absolute levels of each hormone has no effect on whether or not a patient develops postpartum blues; rather, the larger the change prepartum and postpartum, the more likely the person is to develop postpartum blues.[12] A second theory is that it is caused by "a biological system underlying mammalian mother-infant attachment behavior, regulated primarily by the hormone oxytocin."[11] Supporting evidence for this second hypothesis has been shown in rodents that have had their oxytocin-producing cells removed and then had less maternal behaviors.[13]

Postpartum Depression

Postpartum depression most typically emerges within the first 1 to 3 months after delivery but can occur anytime during the first year after delivery and unlike postpartum blues, requires intervention. Sometimes, symptoms start during pregnancy and worsen after delivery. Postpartum depression is clinically indistinguishable from depression during other periods in one's life. The *Diagnostic and Statistical Manual of Mental Disorders*, 5th edition, classifies perinatal depression as a major depressive disorder and describes symptoms as[10]:

- Feeling sad or having a depressed mood
- Loss of interest or pleasure in activities once enjoyed
- Changes in appetite
- Trouble sleeping or sleeping too much
- Loss of energy or increased fatigue
- Increase in purposeless physical activity (eg, inability to sit still, pacing, hand-wringing) or slowed movements or speech (these actions must be severe enough to be observable by others)
- Feeling worthless or guilty
- Difficulty thinking, concentrating, or making decisions
- Thoughts of death or suicide
- Crying for "no reason"
- Lack of interest in the baby, not feeling bonded to the baby, or feeling anxious about/around the baby
- Feelings of being a bad parent
- Fear of harming the baby or oneself

Five symptoms must be present every day for at least 2 weeks and must represent a change from prior functioning.[10] A few mnemonics to remember some of the symptoms to ask about are SIGECAPS and DEPRESSION.[14]

- Depressed mood
- Energy loss/fatigue
- Pleasure lost
- Retardation (psychomotor) or excitation
- Eating changed (appetite/weight)
- Sleep changed
- Suicidal thoughts
- I am a failure (loss of confidence/feelings of worthlessness)
- No concentration

There are a variety of other comorbid mood disorders often associated with postpartum depression. Postpartum anxiety most typically presents within 3 months of delivery with 75% of patients with postpartum depression also developing postpartum anxiety.[15] Panic attacks or hypochondriasis may also develop, sometimes within just a few days of delivery. Postpartum obsessive-compulsive disorder may also develop: up to 75% of patients with a history of obsessive-compulsive disorder have a recurrence following childbirth that typically lasts for at least 6 months.[16] The most commonly reported obsessions were aggression and contamination, whereas the most commonly reported compulsions were cleaning/washing and checking.[12] Posttraumatic stress disorder was present in 1 in 10 after delivery but present in up to 30% whom had complications during their pregnancy or delivery.[7]

Postpartum Psychosis

Postpartum psychosis is the most severe form of a postpartum psychiatric illness and is potentially deadly.[7] It most typically occurs with the first 48 to 72 hours after delivery but can be seen later. It closely resembles a rapidly evolving manic or mixed episode of bipolar illness.[8] The earliest symptoms are restlessness, irritability, and insomnia. Then, a rapidly shifting depressed and elated mood occurs, disorientation, confusion, delusional beliefs (usually centered on newborn), and hallucinations may occur that tell patients to hurt herself or their newborn.[8] A patient with a history of bipolar disorder is 40% more likely to develop postpartum psychosis. Ten percent of cases result in suicide or infanticide.[12]

Although it is difficult to imagine someone taking their life in what people often view as a happy life event, during the last decade suicide attempts during and after pregnancy have tripled in the United States, whereas other causes of maternal mortality decline.[18] Some of this increase is believed to be caused by improvements in appropriate classification of maternal deaths.[19] Prevalence of suicidal ideation ranges from 2% to 5% among women seeking obstetric care.[15] Suicide also remains a leading cause of mortality in the postpartum period and accounts for 20% of maternal deaths in the first year after birth[20] with self-harm risk peaking at 6 to 12 months postpartum. The patients at greatest risk for self-harm included white patients,[15] younger patients,[21] and patients that had a pregnancy loss.[22] More than 60% whom took their own life had not seen a mental health care provider in the month leading up to their death but had in the year before their death.[10] Worldwide prevalence of suicide attempts was 680 per 100,000 during pregnancy and 210 per 100,000 during the first year postpartum.[23] Some studies report that suicide attempts are lower in pregnancy compared with prepregnancy and postpartum, as much as six times lower than in the postnatal period.[24] Other studies, however, have found higher rate of suicide and suicide attempts in the perinatal period indicating that pregnancy is not protective of suicide as previously thought.[25] Prevalence was found to be highest in the first trimester (4.4%) and lower in the second and third trimesters (2.9%).[21] A chart review of female patients hospitalized over a 1-year period in South Africa found that 33% were pregnant at the time of their suicide attempt.[26] Among pregnancy-related mental health deaths in the United States (including suicide and overdose) three-quarters have a history of depression and more than two-thirds have a history (past or current) of substance use disorder.[27]

Paternal perinatal depression is also documented during pregnancy and the postpartum period. Rather than low mood, depressed fathers tend to experience extreme self-criticism, restlessness, increased irritability, and aggression.[28] Depression in new fathers sometimes leads to substance use disorders, food behavior disorders, and lack of impulse control.[28] There are no diagnostic criteria or validated screening tools at this time that specifically address paternal perinatal depression.[28]

INCIDENCE

Postpartum blues occurs in up to 85% of patients during the first 2 weeks after delivery.[5] Perinatal depression, however, has a prepandemic incidence of 12% of all pregnant or postpartum patients in a given year.[29] These numbers vary greatly based on many factors, such as socioeconomic status, education, and ethnicity. For instance, in low income and pregnant or parenting teenagers the incidence is 40% to 60%.[15] In the United States one in seven has been the accepted incidence for postpartum depression for several years.[30–33] With 4 million births each year in the United States this means that 600,000 diagnoses of postpartum depression occur each year. Adding in patients that miscarry or have still births that may also develop depressive symptoms, this can increase diagnoses to almost 1 million diagnoses per year.[17] About 25% of depressive episodes that are identified after delivery actually began before pregnancy and about 30% during pregnancy.[34] Patients with a history of depression that discontinued antidepressants before pregnancy were 68% more likely to have a relapse of depression during pregnancy than patients that did not discontinue their medications before pregnancy.[35] Paternal depression occurs in up to 25% of first time fathers but is up to 50% if their partner has postpartum depression.[28] Twenty-two percent of fathers had depression and anxiety at some point in the first year postpartum.[36,37] Postpartum psychosis occurs in 1 to 3 per 1000 postpartum patients.[12]

Perinatal depression is the most underdiagnosed pregnancy complication in the United States.[38] Perinatal mood disorders are a global health concern because tens, if not hundreds, of millions of patients are diagnosed annually.[12]

- Canada[39]: postpartum depression—23% overall, 30% younger than age 25, older than 30% also had a depressive disorder or mood disorder before pregnancy
- United Kingdom[40]: postpartum depression—1 in 10 overall, 1 in 8 antenatally, 25% still have symptoms after baby turns age 1
- Australia[41]: postpartum depression—1 in 5 do not receive proper prenatal and postnatal follow-up screenings, 40% had symptoms that started during pregnancy
- Philippines[42]: postpartum depression—16.4% at 6 weeks postpartum
- South America[43]: postpartum depression is more common in South America than in higher income countries

The COVID-19 pandemic increased the incidence of perinatal mood disorders around the world. One study showed an increase from 15% to 20% to 36% during pregnancy and after delivery patients were four times more likely to experience significant psychiatric symptoms. Those with preexisting mental health diagnoses were two to four times more likely to develop significant symptoms of depression, anxiety, or posttraumatic stress disorder.[44] Another study showed an increase from 29% to 72% of moderate to high levels of anxiety during pregnancy or after delivery.[45] During the pandemic patients experienced decreased social and emotional support, and unanticipated changes to care plans,[46] birthing experiences, and delivery of infant care, all of which may help explain the increases in perinatal mood disorders.[47,48]

RISK FACTORS

There do not seem to be specific risk factors predisposing one to postpartum blues; however, psychiatric history, stress, cultural context, breastfeeding, and parity may influence whether or not postpartum blues become postpartum depression.[49] Cheryl Beck[50] has created the Postpartum Depression Predictors Inventory, which is a list of 13 risk factors for developing perinatal depression.

Postpartum Depression Predictors Inventory
- Depression during pregnancy is the strongest predictor
- Prenatal anxiety
- Prior history of depression
- Postpartum blues
- Recent stressful life events
- Inadequate social supports
- Poor marital relationship
- Low self-esteem
- Childcare stress
- Difficult infant temperament
- Single marital status
- Unintended pregnancy
- Lower family income

Other perinatal depression risk factors include[51,52]

- There may be none
- Premenstrual syndrome[53]
- Premenstrual dysphoric disorder[54]
- Psychosocial stress
- Multiparity
- Fewer prenatal appointments
- Giving birth in winter[55]
- Pregnancy and delivery complications, such as hyperemesis gravidarum and postpartum hemorrhage[56]
- Infant sleeping problems[57]
- Tobacco use or recently quitting[58]

Perinatal depression protective factors include

- Strong social support[52]
- Exclusive breastfeeding[59]
- Nondepressed partner[60]

Perinatal suicide and suicidal behavior risk factors are similar to those of the general population.[61,62]

- Younger age
- Limited education

- Unmarried
- Marital dissatisfaction
- History of childhood trauma[63]
- Intimate partner violence[64]
- Psychiatric comorbidity[65]
- Financial instability
- Sickness of new baby[66]

Protective factors include

- Good social support[67]
- Cohabitation with partner[68]

PREVENTION AND INTERVENTION STRATEGIES
Prevention

By using the previously mentioned risk factors to identify patients at highest risk for developing perinatal mood disorders more intensive monitoring, services, and interventions can be offered to prevent a perinatal mood disorder from developing.[69] For patients with a history of depression some studies have shown benefit of prophylactic antidepressant therapy after delivery.[70]

Screening recommendations

Patients may be embarrassed to discuss their symptoms, fear being judged, think their symptoms are normal, or have poor mental health awareness. Screening for perinatal mental health disorders and intervening when necessary is important because of the potential adverse effects of untreated mood disorders on the mother, child, and entire family unit.[41] Untreated perinatal mental health disorders place the developing children at a disadvantage right from their birth, causing the cycle of disparity to become a vicious cycle to repeat across generations.[71] Many studies have shown that when left untreated these mental health disorders can lead to impaired mother-infant bonding and breastfeeding,[5] and emotional, behavioral, cognitive, and interpersonal problems later in life for the children.[72] Infants can develop attachment disorder,[73] oppositional defiant disorder, or attention-deficit disorder; have developmental delays at 1 year of age with poor cognitive, motor, and language development, poor physical growth, and poor academic performance; and lower immunization rates throughout childhood.[74–76]

Despite being evidence based[3,77] and recommended by many medical societies including the US Preventive Services Task Force (USPSTF),[78] American College of Obstetricians and Gynecologists (ACOG),[79] American Academy of Family Physicians (AAFP),[80] American Academy of Pediatrics (AAP),[81] American Medical Association, Association of Women's Health, Obstetric and Neonatal Nurses, American College of Nurse Midwives, and the National Institute for Healthcare Excellence,[82] screening is not yet universal.[83] According to the USPSTF screening programs should only be conducted when there are significant and effective treatment and follow-up options available. The Canadian Task Force on Preventive Health Care recommends "against instrument-based depression screening using a questionnaire with cut-off score to distinguish 'screen positive' and 'screen negative' *administered to* all individuals *during pregnancy and the postpartum period.*" The recommendation assumes that as a part of usual care, providers will ask about and be attentive to the mental health and well-being of their patients.[84]

ACOG recommends that screening for perinatal depression and anxiety "take place at least once during the perinatal period using a validated screening tool. If a patient is screened during pregnancy additional screening should occur postpartum."[67] AAP recommends screening for perinatal depression at all infant well visits until 6 months of age.[68] The primary care provider (PCP) might be the first clinical contact after delivery for the parent suffering with a perinatal mood disorder. If the PCP is the infant's provider they would not be treating the parent but as recommended would still screen the parent and should collaborate with the parent's provider on treatment. The pregnancy care provider might not see the postpartum patient for up to 6 weeks after delivery, although newer recommendations are to have a 1- to 2-week postpartum visit for all patients, not just patients that had a high-risk pregnancy. If the pregnancy care provider suspects or diagnoses perinatal mood disorders they may initiate treatment, collaborate with other providers on treatment, or refer treatment to mental health providers and the patient's PCP. In the case of some family physicians the infant and mother might have the same PCP, and the family physician might also be the pregnancy care provider so continuity of care and collaboration only needs to be done with a mental health care provider. Collaborative, collocated, and integrated models of mental health care services in the primary care office are promoted by the AAFP and AAP. This approach can provide immediate services when a screen is positive.

Collaborative management uses a team approach. Members of the team should include the PCP; mental health specialist, such as a therapist; and a care manager. The entire team works together to treat the patient using six components of care[85]:

- Reliable screening tool
- Systemic follow-up and monitoring
- Evidence-based guidelines for treatment modification
- Plans for relapse prevention once patients "graduate" from collaborative care management
- Care manager roles to maintain patient contact, education, and coordination of care
- Psychiatrist consultant to oversee care managers and make treatment plans as needed

Screening tools
The following screening tools are used[66,86,87]: Edinburgh Postnatal Depression Scale,[88] Patient Health Questionnaire-9,[89] Postpartum Depression Screening Scale, and Beck Depression Inventory I or II.

- Edinburgh Postnatal Depression Scale
  - Most commonly used
  - Available in 50 different languages
  - 10 questions that are health literacy appropriate
  - Less than 5 minutes to complete
  - Excludes constitutional symptoms of depression, which are common in pregnancy and postpartum period (eg, changes in sleep habits and appetite)
  - Sensitivity 59% to 100%; specificity 49% to 100%
- Patient Health Questionnaire-9
  - 9 questions
  - Less than 5 minutes to complete
  - Sensitivity 75%; specificity 90%
- Postpartum Depression Screening Scale
  - 35 questions
  - 5 to 10 minutes to complete
  - Sensitivity 91% to 94%; specificity 72% to 98%

- Beck Depression Inventory I or II
  - 21 questions
  - 5 to 10 minutes to complete
  - Beck I: sensitivity 47.6% to 82%; specificity 85.9% to 89%
  - Beck II: sensitivity 56% to 57%; specificity 77% to 88%

Interventions

Improving access to care and using telehealth,[90] collaborative and integrative mental health treatment approaches are intervention strategies specifically recommended to reduce the risks of adverse effects to the family unit. Family-focused approaches that provide emotional support and parenting support to both parents are often most helpful. Incorporating the father into treatment can help combat stigma around perinatal mood disorder diagnoses and help any potential gendered parenting roles that they may be struggling with and cultivate support networks that are often lacking.[28] Family-focused approaches include

- Internet communities
- In-home support visits
- Nurse-family partnerships
- Community health workers
- Telephone-based peer support
- E-therapy
- Group workshops

It is also important to think about breastfeeding support, prenatal and postpartum education classes, parenting classes, exercise, and diet, and any other supports/services that the family may need.[5,91] Many health systems, health departments, and organizations have "warm lines" for perinatal mental health that providers can call for assistance with patient cases. There are also patient help lines for patients in crisis that can be used to increase accessibility to mental health providers. Postpartum Support International[92] is an organization established in 1987 with the mission of "promoting awareness, prevention, and treatment of mental health issues related to childbearing." They provide free consultation services for health care professionals, a provider directory, trainings, and help lines for patients. The National Maternal Mental Health Hotline[93] provided by the US Department of Health Resources and Services Administration is another hotline available to patients 24/7 that is free and confidential. There are promotional materials available on their Web site to have available to give to patients that might need it; including it in all preconception counseling, prenatal counseling, and postpartum counseling materials should be a best practice for all pregnancy care providers.

Behavioral management

Cognitive behavioral therapy (CBT) is a structured psychological treatment based on several core principles: (1) psychological problems are in part because of unhelpful ways of thinking, (2) on learned patterns of unhelpful behavior, and (3) that people with psychological problems can learn coping mechanisms to help relieve their symptoms. CBT usually involves changing ones thinking and behavioral patterns with various techniques and involves making a plan with the therapist plus doing "homework" outside of sessions.[94] CBT is the first-line therapy for perinatal depression and is as effective, or more effective than medication.[95,96] One study showed that even a 1-day online workshop on CBT (plus treatment as usual) was sufficient to improve postpartum depression and anxiety and mother-infant bonding and social support.[97] Interpersonal therapy has also been shown to be effective for perinatal mood disorders and improving the quality of interpersonal relationships and social functioning. This type of therapy is time-limited, focused, and addresses interpersonal deficits, social isolation, involvement in unfulfilling relationships, helps patients understand unresolved grief, and helps with difficult life transitions. It addresses maladaptive thoughts and behaviors only as they apply to interpersonal relationships and aims to change relationship patterns that the patient is currently involved in, whereas CBT also addresses past relationships, personality traits, and is more directive.[98]

Pharmacologic management

If nonpharmacologic interventions are inadequate beginning pharmacologic management with selective serotonin reuptake inhibitors (SSRIs) is favored. ACOG recommends using one medication at a higher dose rather than using multiple medications to limit risks. It is also best practice to use a medication that the patient has previously had success with, if one exists.[99] Providers must assess the risk of inadequately treated illness and potential adverse effects of medication with respect to pregnancy and infant outcomes. There are many resources to look up the risks of medication during pregnancy and lactation including textbooks, online resources, and phone apps. The Food and Drug Administration (FDA) new revision of the Pregnancy and Lactation Labeling Rule that occurred in 2015 gives much more information now than just a letter grade of each medication. It gives clinical summaries, comprehensive information on potential risks and benefits, data on clinical experience, animal data, and risks of untreated illness.[100]

Recent data from 2019 to 2022 show that SSRI exposure does not increase risk of major congenital malformations. However, they are associated with a low absolute risk of preeclampsia, postpartum hemorrhage, preterm delivery, persistent pulmonary hypertension of the newborn, and neonatal intensive care unit admissions when compared with untreated perinatal depression.[101] However, another large cohort study of more than 100,000 pregnant women with depression did not find an association between SSRIs and preeclampsia but did find an association with preeclampsia and serotonin-norepinephrine reuptake inhibitors and tricyclic antidepressants when used as monotherapy during pregnancy.[102] In contrast to the 2019 to 2022 data, a large meta-analysis showed that the risk of preterm birth was no longer significant when compared with women with untreated perinatal depression.[103] Preferred SSRIs to use in pregnancy are sertraline, citalopram, escitalopram, and fluoxetine because of low risk of birth defects. Paroxetine is not recommended to be used in pregnancy because of risk of cardiac malformations.[104]

In 2019, the FDA approved brexanolone, an injection for intravenous use for treatment of postpartum depression. Brexanolone is the first medication to receive FDA approval for postpartum depression[105] after three clinical trials established its efficacy and safety.[106] There are potential serious risks associated with this medication, however, so it is only available through Risk Evaluation and Mitigation Strategy; patients are only able to get the medication at health care facilities at which they can be monitored while receiving an intravenous infusion for 60 continuous hours.

Electroconvulsive therapy is used for severe cases when all other treatments have failed.[107]

CLINICS CARE POINTS

- Postpartum blues occurs during the first 2 weeks postpartum and although symptoms are unsettling and unpredictable, they do not impair function or only cause mild dysfunction and it is never accompanied by suicidal ideation.

- 12% of all pregnant or postpartum patients in a given year experience postpartum depression.
- All pregnant and postpartum patients should be screened for perinatal mood disorders with validated screening tools, such as the Edinburgh Postnatal Depression Scale, Patient Health Questionnaire-9, Postpartum Depression Screening Scale, or Beck Depression Inventory I or II.
- Intervention should be collaborative with integrative mental health treatment approaches using family-focused care and providing emotional and parenting support to both parents. Providing other types of support, education, services, and resources can also be an important part of care.
- Pharmacologic management should be considered when other interventions have been inadequate.

DISCLOSURE

No disclosures or conflicts of interest.

REFERENCES

1. Waqas A, Raza N, Lodhi HW, et al. Psychosocial factors of antenatal anxiety and depression in Pakistan: is social support a mediator? PLoS One 2015;10(1): e0116510.
2. Lin B, Kalilush P, Conradt E, et al. Intergenerational transmission of emotion dysregulation: Part I. Psychopathology, self-injury, and parasympathetic responsivity among pregnant women. Dev Psychopathol 2019;31:817–31.
3. Waqas A, Koukab A, Meraj H, et al. Screening programs for common maternal mental health disorders among perinatal women: report of the systematic review of evidence. BMC Psychiatry 2022;22(1):54.
4. Gelaye B, Rondon MB, Araya R, et al. Epidemiology of maternal depression, risk factors, and child outcomes in low-income and middle-income countries. Lancet Psychiatry 2016;3(10):973–82.
5. Newman DM, Boyarsky M, Mayo D. Postpartum depression. JAAPA 2022;35(4): 54–5. PMID: 35348542.
6. Palladino CL, Singh V, Campbell J, et al. Homicide and suicide during the perinatal period: findings from the National Violent Death Reporting System. Obstet Gynecol 2011;118(5):1056–63.
7. Bauer A, Parsonage M, Knapp M, et al. The costs of perinatal mental health problems. LSE Cent Ment Heal 2014;1–44. Available at:.
8. Jones I, Shakespeare J. Postnatal depression. BMJ 2014;349:g4500.
9. Miller LJ. Postpartum depression. JAMA 2002;287(6):762–5.
10. American Psychiatric Association. Diagnostic and Statistical Manual of Mental Disorders. 5th edition. Washington, DC: American Psychiatric Association; 2013.
11. Miller LJ, Girgis C, Gupta R. Depression and related disorders during the female reproductive cycle. Women's Health 2009;5(5):577–87.
12. Harris B, Lovett L, Newcombe RG, et al. Maternity blues and major endocrine changes. BMJ 1994;308:949–53.
13. Saltzman W, Maestripieri D. The neuroendocrinology of primate maternal behavior. Prog Neuropsychopharmacol Biol Psychiatry 2011;35(5):1192–204. Epub 2010 Oct 1. PMID: 20888383; PMCID: PMC3072435.

14. Blenkiron P. A mnemonic for depression. BMJ 2006;332(7540):551. PMCID: PMC1388172.
15. Miller ES, Hoxha D, Wisner KL, et al. The impact of perinatal depression on the evolution of anxiety and obsessive-compulsive symptoms. Arch Womens Ment Health 2015;18(3):457–61.
16. Miller ES, Hoxha D, Wisner KL, et al. Obsessions and compulsions in post-partum women without obsessive compulsive disorder. J Womens Health (Larchmt) 2015;24(10):825–30.
17. Andersen LB, Melvaer LB, Videbech P, et al. Risk factors for developing post-traumatic stress disorder following childbirth: a systematic review. Acta Obstet Gynecol Scand. 2012. 91(11):1261-1272.
18. Chin K, Wendt A, Bennett IM, et al. Suicide and maternal mortality. Curr Psychiatry Rep 2022;24(4):239–75. Epub 2022 Apr 2. PMID: 35366195; PMCID: PMC8976222.
19. Langdon MDK. Statistics on postpartum depression: postpartum depression resources. [online] PostpartumDepression.org. 2022. Available at: https://www.postpartumdepression.org/resources/statistics/. Accessed 16 May 2022.
20. Kendig S, Keats JP, Hoffman MC, et al. Consensus bundle on maternal mental health: perinatal depression and anxiety. J Obstet Gynecol Neonatal Nurs 2017; 46:272–81.
21. Hope H, Pierce M, Osam CS, et al. Self-harm risk in pregnancy: recurrent-event survival analysis using UK primary care data. Br J Psychiatry 2022;221(4): 621–7.
22. Gavin NI, Gaynes BN, Lohr KN, et al. Perinatal depression: a systematic review of prevalence and incidence. Obstet Gynecol 2005;106(5 Pt 1):1071–83.
23. Mutiso SK, Murage A, Mukaindo AM. Prevalence of positive depression screen among post miscarriage women: a cross sectional study. BMC Psychiatry 2018; 18(1):32. PMID: 29402255; PMCID: PMC5799918.
24. Rao WW, Yang Y, Ma TJ, et al. Worldwide prevalence of suicide attempt in pregnant and postpartum women: a meta-analysis of observational studies. Soc Psychiatry Psychiatr Epidemiol 2021;56(5):711–20. Epub 2020 Nov 16. PMID: 33191455.
25. Appleby L. Suicide during pregnancy and in the first postnatal year. BMJ 1991; 302(6769):137–40. PMCID: PMC1668816.
26. Kitsantas P, Aljoudi SM, Adams AR, et al. Prevalence and correlates of suicidal behaviors during pregnancy: evidence from the National Survey on Drug Use and Health. Arch Womens Ment Health 2021;24(3):473–81. Epub 2020 Nov 21. PMID: 33222035.
27. Vawda NBM. Suicide attempts during pregnancy in South Africa. S Afr J Psychiatr 2018;24:1154. PMID: 30263220; PMCID: PMC6138131.
28. Trost SL, Beauregard JL, Smoots AN, et al. Preventing pregnancy-related mental health deaths: insights from 14 US Maternal Mortality Review Committees, 2008-17. Health Aff (Millwood) 2021;40(10):1551–9.
29. Chavis AT. Paternal perinatal depression in modern-day fatherhood. Pediatr Rev 2022;43(10):539–48. PMID: 36180540.
30. Isaacs M. Community care networks for depression in low-income communities and communities of color: a review of the literature. Washington, DC: Howard University School of Social Work and the National Alliance of Multiethnic Behavioral Health Associations; 2004.
31. Hahn-Holbrook J, Cornwell-Hinrichs T, Anaya I. Economic and health predictors of national postpartum depression prevalence: a systematic review, meta-

analysis, and meta-regression of 291 studies from 56 countries. Front Psychiatry 2018;8.

32. Shorey S, Chee CYI, Ng ED, et al. Prevalence and incidence of postpartum depression among healthy mothers: a systematic review and meta-analysis. J Psychiatr Res 2018;104:235–48.

33. Fawcett EJ, Fairbrother N, Cox ML, et al. The prevalence of anxiety disorders during pregnancy and the postpartum period. J Clin Psychiatry 2019;80.

34. Wisner KL, Sit DK, McShea MC, et al. Onset timing, thoughts of self-harm, and diagnoses in postpartum women with screen-positive depression findings. JAMA Psychiatry 2013;70:490–8.

35. Goodman JH. Paternal postpartum depression, its relationship to maternal postpartum depression, and implications for family health. J Adv Nurs 2004;45(1): 26–35.

36. Rossi NM, Radney L. Diagnosis and management of perinatal depression. Nurs Womens Health 2022;26(4):318–30. Epub 2022 Jun 15. PMID: 35714763.

37. Dennis CL, Marini F, Dol J, et al. Paternal prevalence and risk factors for comorbid depression and anxiety across the first 2 years postpartum: a nationwide Canadian cohort study. Depress Anxiety 2022;39(3):233–45.

38. Facts, Stats Maternal Mental Health in Canada. The Vanier Institute of the Family/L'Institut Vanier de la famille. 2022. Available at: https://vanierinstitute.ca/. Accessed May 16, 2022.

39. Howard LM, Khalifeh H. Perinatal mental health: a review of progress and challenges. World Psychiatry 2020;19(3):313–27.

40. Australian Institute of Health and Welfare. Experience of perinatal depression: data from the 2010 Australian national infant feeding survey. Information paper. Cat. No. PHE 161. Canberra: AIHW; 2012.

41. Labrague LJ, McEnroe-Petitte D, Tsaras K, et al. Predictors of postpartum depression and the utilization of postpartum depression services in rural areas in the Philippines. Perspect Psychiatr Care 2020;56(2):308–15.

42. Rondon MB. Perinatal mental health around the world: priorities for research and service development in South America. Bjpsych Int 2020;17(4):85–7.

43. Liu CH, Erdei C, Mittal L. Risk factors for depression, anxiety, and PTSD symptoms in perinatal women during the COVID-19 pandemic. Psychiatry Res 2021; 295:113552.

44. Davenport MH, Meyer S, Meah VL, et al. Moms are not OK: COVID-19 and maternal mental health. Front Glob Womens Health 2020;1:1.

45. Shuman CJ, Peahl AF, Pareddy N, et al. Postpartum depression and associated risk factors during the COVID-19 pandemic. BMC Res Notes 2022;15(1):102.

46. Experiences of peripartum women during the COVID-19 pandemic. Matern Child Health J 2022;26(1):102–9.

47. Safi-Keykaleh M, Aliakbari F, Safarpour H, et al. Prevalence of postpartum depression in women amid the COVID-19 pandemic: a systematic review and meta-analysis. Int J Gynaecol Obstet 2022;157(2):240–7. Epub 2022 Feb 28. PMID: 35122433; PMCID: PMC9087783.

48. Hapgood CC, Elkind GS, Wright JJ. Maternity blues: phenomena and relationship to later postpartum depression. Aust N Z J Psychiatry 1988;22:299–306.

49. Beck CT. Predictors of postpartum depression: an update. Nurs Res 2001;50(5): 275–85.

50. Oliveira TA, Luzetti GGCM, Rosalém MMA, et al. Screening of perinatal depression using the Edinburgh Postpartum Depression Scale. Rev Bras Ginecol Obstet 2022;44(5):452–7. Epub 2022 Mar 4. PMID: 35253138.

51. Munk-Olsen T, Liu X, Madsen KB, et al. Postpartum depression: a developed and validated model predicting individual risk in new mothers. Transl Psychiatry 2022;12(1):419. PMCID: PMC9525696.

52. Yücesoy H, Erbi LN. Relationship of premenstrual syndrome with postpartum depression and mother-infant bonding. Perspect Psychiatr Care 2022;58(3): 1112–20. Epub 2021 Jul 7. PMID: 34231233.

53. Pereira D, Pessoa AR, Madeira N, et al. Association between premenstrual dysphoric disorder and perinatal depression: a systematic review. Arch Womens Ment Health 2022;25(1):61–70. Epub 2021 Aug 26. PMID: 34436653.

54. Tung TH, Jiesisibieke D, Xu Q, et al. Relationship between seasons and postpartum depression: a systematic review and meta-analysis of cohort studies. Brain Behav 2022;12(6):e2583. Epub 2022 May 3. PMID: 35502646; PMCID: PMC9226811.

55. Wang K, Qiu J, Meng L, et al. Postpartum hemorrhage and postpartum depressive symptoms: a retrospective cohort study. Depress Anxiety 2022;39(3): 246–53. Epub 2022 Feb 15. PMID: 35167153.

56. Škodová Z, Kelčíková S, Maskálová E, et al. Infant sleep and temperament characteristics in association with maternal postpartum depression. Midwifery 2022; 105:103232. Epub 2021 Dec 21. PMID: 34971869.

57. Yook V, Yoo J, Han K, et al. Association between pre-pregnancy tobacco smoking and postpartum depression: a nationwide cohort study. J Affect Disord 2022;316:56–62. Epub 2022 Aug 5. PMID: 35940375.

58. Xia M, Luo J, Wang J, et al. Association between breastfeeding and postpartum depression: a meta-analysis. J Affect Disord 2022;308:512–9. Epub 2022 Apr 20. PMID: 35460745.

59. Mezulis AH, Hyde JS, Clark R. Father involvement moderates the effect of maternal depression during a child's infancy on child behavior problems in kindergarten. J Fam Psychol 2004;18(4):575–88.

60. MGH Center for Women's Mental Health. Postpartum psychiatric disorders - MGH Center for Women's Mental Health. 2022 [online] Available at: https://womensmentalhealth.org/specialty-clinics/postpartum-psychiatric-disorders/. Accessed 8 April 2022.

61. Levey EJ, Rondon MB, Sanchez S, et al. Suicide risk assessment: examining transitions in suicidal behaviors among pregnant women in Perú. Arch Womens Ment Health 2019;22(1):65–73. Epub 2018 Jul 3. PMID: 29971552; PMCID: PMC6571105.

62. Meurk C, Wittenhagen L, Lucke J, et al. Suicidal behaviours in the peripartum period: a systematic scoping review of data linkage studies. Arch Womens Ment Health 2021;24(4):579–93. Epub 2021 Mar 19. PMID: 33742281.

63. Ammerman RT, Scheiber FA, Peugh JL, et al. Interpersonal trauma and suicide attempts in low-income depressed mothers in home visiting. Child Abuse Negl 2019;97:104126. Epub 2019 Aug 29. PMID: 31473381; PMCID: PMC6773481.

64. Campbell J, Matoff-Stepp S, Velez ML, et al. Pregnancy-associated deaths from homicide, suicide, and drug overdose: review of research and the intersection with intimate partner violence. J Womens Health (Larchmt) 2021;30(2):236–44. PMID: 33295844; PMCID: PMC8020563.

65. Jago CA, Crawford SG, Gill SJ, et al. Mental health and maternal mortality-when new life doesn't bring joy. J Obstet Gynaecol Can 2021;43(1):67–73.e1. Epub 2020 Jul 4. PMID: 32978085.

66. Belete H, Misgan E. Suicidal behaviour in postnatal mothers in northwestern Ethiopia: a cross-sectional study. BMJ Open 2019;9(9):e027449. PMID: 31530587; PMCID: PMC6756460.

67. Martini J, Bauer M, Lewitzka U, et al. Predictors and outcomes of suicidal ideation during peripartum period. J Affect Disord 2019;257:518–26. Epub 2019 Jul 5. PMID: 31323593.

68. Kubota C, Inada T, Shiino T, et al. The risk factors predicting suicidal ideation among perinatal women in Japan. Front Psychiatry 2020;11:441. PMID: 32499731; PMCID: PMC7242750.

69. Dennis CL. Psychosocial and psychological interventions for prevention of postnatal depression: systematic review. BMJ 2005;331(7507):15.

70. Wisner KL, Perel JM, Peindl KS, et al. Prevention of postpartum depression: a pilot randomized clinical trial. Am J Psychiatry 2004;161(7):1290–2.

71. Zafar S, Sikander S, Haq Z, et al. Integrating maternal psychosocial well-being into a child-development intervention: the five-pillars approach. Ann N Y Acad Sci 2014;1308:107–17.

72. Christaki V, Ismirnioglou I, Katrali A, et al. Postpartum depression and ADHD in the offspring: systematic review and meta-analysis. J Affect Disord 2022;318: 314–30. Epub 2022 Sep 9. PMID: 36096371.

73. Martins C, Gaffan EA. Effects of early maternal depression on patterns of infant-mother attachment: a meta-analytic investigation. J Child Psychol Psychiatry 2000;41:737–46.

74. Burger M, Hoosain M, Einspieler C, et al. Maternal perinatal mental health and infant and toddler neurodevelopment: evidence from low and middle-income countries. A systematic review. J Affect Disord 2020;268:158–72.

75. Cummings EM, Davies PT. Maternal depression and child development. J Child Psychol Psychiatry 1994;35:73–122.

76. Kingston D, Tough S, Whitfield H. Prenatal and postpartum maternal psychological distress and infant development: a systematic review. Child Psychiatry Hum Dev 2012;43:683–714.

77. Morrell CJ, Warner R, Slade P, et al. Psychological interventions for postnatal depression: cluster randomised trial and economic evaluation. The PoNDER trial. Health Technol Assess (Rockv) 2009;13(30):1–53.

78. Siu AL, US Preventive Services Task Force (USPSTF), Bibbins-Domingo K, et al. Screening for depression in adults: US Preventive Services Task Force Recommendation Statement. JAMA 2016;315(4):380–7.

79. ACOG Committee Opinion No. 757: screening for perinatal depression. Obstet Gynecol 2018;132(5):e208–12.

80. Langan R, Goodbred AJ. Identification and management of peripartum depression. Am Fam Physician 2016;93(10):852–8.

81. Earls MF, Yogman MW. Mattson G, et al. Incorporating recognition and management of perinatal depression into pediatric practice. Pediatrics 2019;143(1): e20183259.

82. Milgrom J, Gemmill AW. International Approaches to Perinatal Mental Health Screening as a Public Health Priority, . Identifying perinatal depression and anxiety: evidence-based practice in screening, psychosocial assessment and management. Chichester, West Sussex: Wiley-Blackwell; 2015.

83. National Collaborating Center for Mental Health. The NICE guideline on the management and treatment of depression in adults. Updated edition 2010.

84. Depression during pregnancy and the postpartum period. Canadian Task Force on preventive health care 2022. Available at: https://canadiantaskforce.ca/

guidelines/published-guidelines/depression-during-pregnancy-and-the-postpartum-period/. Accessed October 19, 2022.

85. Truitt FE, Pina BJ, Person-Rennell NH, et al. Outcomes for collaborative care versus routine care in the management of postpartum depression. Qual Prim Care 2013;21(3):171–7.

86. Zubaran C, Schumacher M, Roxo MR, et al. Screening tools for postpartum depression: validity and cultural dimensions. Afr J Psychiatry (Johannesbg) 2010;13(5):357–65.

87. Joffres M, Jaramillo A, Dickinson J, et al. Recommendations on screening for depression in adults. CMAJ 2013;185(9):775–82.

88. Cox JL, Holden JM, Sagovsky R. Detection of postnatal depression: development of the 10-item Edinburgh Postnatal Depression Scale. Br J Psychiatry 1987;150(6):782–6.

89. Spitzer RL, Kroenke K, Williams JBW, the Patient Health Questionnaire Study Group. Validity and utility of a self-report version of PRIME-MD: the PHQ Primary Care Study. JAMA 1999;282:1737–44.

90. Osborne LM, Kimmel MC, Surkan PJ. The crisis of perinatal mental health in the age of COVID-19. Matern Child Health J 2021;25(3):349–52.

91. Dennis CL, Dowswell T. Psychosocial and psychological interventions for preventing postpartum depression. Cochrane Database Syst Rev 2013;2: CD001134.

92. Postpartum Support - PSI. Postpartum support - PSI 2014. Available at: https://www.postpartum.net/.

93. National Maternal Mental Health Hotline | MCHB. mchb.hrsa.gov. Available at: https://mchb.hrsa.gov/national-maternal-mental-health-hotline. Accessed October 1, 2022.

94. American Psychological Association. What is cognitive behavioral therapy? Am Psychol Assoc 2017. Available at: https://www.apa.org/ptsd-guideline/patients-and-families/cognitive-behavioral.

95. Gautam M, Tripathi A, Deshmukh D, et al. Cognitive behavioral therapy for depression. Indian J Psychiatry 2020;62(Suppl 2):S223–9. Epub 2020 Jan 17. PMID: 32055065; PMCID: PMC7001356.

96. Li Z, Liu Y, Wang J, et al. Effectiveness of cognitive behavioural therapy for perinatal depression: a systematic review and meta-analysis. J Clin Nurs 2020; 29(17–18):3170–82. Epub 2020 Jul 15. PMID: 32563204.

97. Rosenberg K. One-day workshop beneficial for postpartum depression. Am J Nurs 2022;122(2):49–50. PMID: 35085151.

98. Weissman MM. Interpersonal psychotherapy: history and future. Am J Psychother 2020;73(1):3–7. Epub 2019 Nov 22. PMID: 31752510.

99. Wisner KL, Parry BL, Piontek CM. Clinical practice. Postpartum depression. N Engl J Med 2002;347(3):194–9.

100. Byrne JJ, Saucedo AM, Spong CY. Evaluation of drug labels following the 2015 pregnancy and lactation labeling rule. JAMA Netw Open 2020;3(8):e2015094.

101. Lebin LG, Novick AM. Selective serotonin reuptake inhibitors (SSRIs) in pregnancy: an updated review on risks to mother, fetus, and child. Curr Psychiatry Rep 2022. https://doi.org/10.1007/s11920-022-01372-x. Epub ahead of print. PMID: 36181572.

102. Palmsten Kristina, Huybrechts Krista Fb, Michels Karin Ba, et al. Antidepressant use and risk for preeclampsia. Epidemiol September 2013;24(5):682–91.

103. Ross LE, Grigoriadis S, Mamisashvili L, et al. Selected pregnancy and delivery outcomes after exposure to antidepressant medication. JAMA Psychiatry 2013; 70(4):436–43.
104. Bérard A, Iessa N, Chaabane S, et al. The risk of major cardiac malformations associated with paroxetine use during the first trimester of pregnancy: a systematic review and meta-analysis. Br J Clin Pharmacol 2016;81(4):589–604.
105. FDA. (2019). FDA approves first treatment for post-partum depression. U.S. Food and Drug Administration. Retrieved October 19, 2022, Available at: https://www.fda.gov/news-events/press-announcements/fda-approves-first-treatment-post-partum-depression
106. Patatanian E, Nguyen DR. Brexanolone: A novel drug for the treatment of post-partum depression. J Pharm Pract 2022;35(3):431–6. Epub 2020 Dec 11. PMID: 33302791.
107. Yonkers KA, Vigod S, Ross LE. Diagnosis, pathophysiology, and management of mood disorders in pregnant and postpartum women. Obstet Gynecol 2011; 117(4):961–77.

Geriatric Depression

Elizabeth Gundersen, MD, FHM[a],*, Benjamin Bensadon, EdM, PhD[b]

KEYWORDS

- Older adults • Geriatric • Depression • Aging • Integrated care

KEY POINTS

- Contrary to common stereotypes, depression is not a normal part of aging.
- Late-life depression is not uncommon but is often underrecognized and undertreated leading to significant morbidity and mortality.
- The bidirectional relationship between late-life depression and concomitant medical illness requires a careful history in order to make an accurate diagnosis of depression.
- Nonpharmacologic geriatric depression treatment is patient-centered and evidence-based.
- Although both pharmacotherapy and psychosocial interventions, or a combination of the two, are considered as the first-line therapy for late-life depression, most data support a combined, biopsychosocial treatment approach provided by an interdisciplinary team.

INTRODUCTION

Late-life depression refers to a major depressive disorder occurring in adults aged 60 years or older. It is a potentially life-threatening problem associated with medical comorbidity, cognitive impairment, disability, both overutilization and underutilization of the health-care system, and suicide.[1] In spite of these risks, depression in older adults is underdiagnosed and undertreated,[2–5] especially among Black and Hispanic men.[6–8]

More than 80% of late-life depression treatment occurs in the primary care setting,[9] where many older adults prefer to address psychosocial issues. It is therefore critical for primary care clinicians to be adept at both recognizing and treating depressive disorders in older adults. Depression is not a normal part of aging, and clinicians should take care not to dismiss the signs and symptoms of depression as merely age-related changes or normal responses to challenging life circumstances or medical problems. At the same time, it is also important to rule out medical conditions before making a diagnosis of depression.

[a] University of Colorado School of Medicine, Mail Stop B178 Academic Office One, 12631 E. 17th Avenue, Aurora, CO 80045, USA; [b] SIMEDHealth, 4343 West Newberry Road, Gainesville, FL 32607, USA
* Corresponding author.
E-mail address: elizabeth.gundersen@cuanschutz.edu

Prim Care Clin Office Pract 50 (2023) 143–158
https://doi.org/10.1016/j.pop.2022.10.010

Historically, either pharmacotherapy or psychotherapy has been considered as the first-line therapy for late-life depression[1] but there is considerable controversy surrounding the utility of antidepressant medications in geriatric depression.[10] The authors present a scoping review of evidence-based approaches to unipolar depression in the primary care setting. As described later, most data support a combined, biopsychosocial treatment approach provided by an interdisciplinary clinical team.

EPIDEMIOLOGY

Ageism (ie, bias based on age)[11] and aging stereotypes lead to assumptions that aging-associated challenges make depression in older adults more prevalent and less treatable in older than younger patients though data reveal the opposite. The prevalence of major depression is actually lower in older adults compared with younger and middle-aged adults.[12] Approximately 5% of community-dwelling older adults have major depression,[13] and most (75%) of them initially present their concerns in a primary care setting. Approximately, 8% to 16% of older persons have clinically significant depressive symptoms that do not meet the standard threshold criteria for major depressive disorder.[13]

Prevalence of major depressive disorders increases with chronic medical comorbidities (ie, multimorbidity), approaching 12% to 30% in patients living in long-term care facilities[14] and as high as 37% after critical care hospitalizations.[15] Indeed, elderly persons with depression typically have at least one concomitant medical comorbidity. Medical conditions associated with high rates of depression include cardiovascular, cerebrovascular, and neurodegenerative disorders as well as cancer.[16] Adults aged 85 years and older may have an increased prevalence of depressive symptoms but this is difficult to estimate because this cohort is often excluded from epidemiologic studies.[17,18]

Suicide

Older adults complete suicide more than any other age demographic in the United States.[19] Depression is the most common diagnosis among older adults who commit suicide. In contrast, younger people who complete suicide most commonly carry diagnoses related to substance abuse and psychosis.[14] Most older persons who complete suicide do so while facing their first depressive episode and about 75% visit a primary care physician in the month preceding the suicide but their symptoms are often unrecognized and untreated.[19–21]

Older adults attempt suicide less frequently than younger people but are more likely to complete their attempts,[22] with White men aged 85 years or older having the highest completion rate.[23] Differentiating medical versus psychological determinants of suicide can be difficult and some data suggest those more seriously ill medically are more likely than healthier patients to attribute their suicide attempt to psychological pain (84% vs 48%).[24]

RISK FACTORS

Risk factors for depression range across biological, physical, psychological, and social factors. They include the following:[15]

- Female sex
- Comorbid medical conditions
- Poorly controlled pain

- Insomnia
- Cognitive impairment
- Impaired functional status
- Social isolation
- Lower socioeconomic status
- Widowed, divorced, or single marital status.

Patients who experience their first depressive episode later in life may be less able to cope and are less likely to have a family history of major mental illness, suggesting genetics plays less of a role in late-life depression than it does in earlier-onset depression.[4,25] Psychosocial stressors such as the death of a loved one may trigger depression. Grief may also mimic depression so patients experiencing adverse life events must be carefully assessed. A notable evolution in the Diagnostic and Statistical Manual of Mental Disorders, fifth edition (DSM-5), is that grief after the death of a loved one is no longer considered exclusionary to making the diagnosis of depression.

Insomnia is a depression risk factor worthy of special emphasis. It is both a risk factor for late-life depression and a presenting symptom for many older adults with depression. In addition, persistent insomnia increases the risk of unremitting depression[26] and the recurrence of depression in remission.[27]

DIAGNOSIS

According to the DSM-5, the diagnosis of major depression requires 5 or more of the following symptoms to be present nearly every day during a 2-week period; one of the symptoms must be either depressed mood or loss of interest or pleasure:[28]

- Depressed mood
- Diminished interest or loss of pleasure in almost all activities
- Significant weight change or appetite disturbance
- Sleep disturbance (insomnia or hypersomnia)
- Psychomotor agitation or retardation
- Fatigue or loss of energy
- Feelings of worthlessness
- Diminished ability to think or concentrate
- Recurrent thoughts of death or suicide.

It is vital that primary care physicians assess their older adult patients for depression, especially during stressful, often seminal life events, in order to ensure timely diagnosis and treatment. Making the diagnosis of late-life depression is challenging and screening must be followed by a careful and comprehensive evaluation in order to avoid improper diagnoses and unnecessary treatments.[29]

The US Preventative Services Task Force recommends depression screening if the resources for further evaluation and management are available, and Medicare Part B covers annual depression screening. The American College of Physicians has advocated for standard behavioral health integration in primary care settings,[30] and the National Academy of Medicine has revealed that without standard integration, evidence-based psychosocial interventions are not delivered.[31]

There are several validated screening instruments available for use in primary care and other settings; a selection of the most commonly used can be found in **Table 1**. All of these scales are considered effective screening tools with high sensitivity and specificity.[32–40]

Screening must be followed by a thorough assessment including a detailed history, physical examination, and laboratory studies. Diagnosing late-life depression is

Table 1
Screening instruments for depression

Screening Instrument	Number of Items	Time to Complete	Scoring
Patient Health Questionnaire 2 (PHQ-2)	2	1 min	≥3 suggests depression
Geriatric Depression Scale (5 item)	5	1 min	≥2 positive answers suggest depression
Patient Health Questionnaire 9 (PHQ-9)	9	5 min	1–4 points = minimal depression, 5–9 points = mild depression, 10–14 points = moderate depression, 15–19 points = moderately severe depression, 20–27 points = severe depression
Cornell Scale for Depression in Dementia	19	5 min with input from caregiver	≥12 suggests depression
Center for Epidemiologic Studies Depression Scale	20	5 min	≥16 suggests depression

complicated. There is some evidence that older adults with depression may present with more somatic complaints than their younger counterparts[41] and may be less likely to describe sadness or guilt. Older adults may have age-related changes such as pale and thinning skin or loss of teeth that can be misinterpreted as depression. As mentioned, they are also more likely to have medical comorbidities and rely on medications that can cause symptoms characteristic of depression (**Table 2**). Therefore, physical illnesses or medication side effects should be excluded before making the diagnosis of depression. Patients should also be asked about alcohol or substance use because these are also associated with depression Other key components of the history are included in table 5.

Suspicion for depression in the setting of concomitant medical illness should be heightened if the patient's mood or physical symptoms seem disproportionate to their underlying disease; if they respond poorly to standard medical treatment; and if they seem unmotivated or disengaged with their care. Patients should be assessed for suicidality and promptly referred to psychiatric care for acute suicidal ideations.

Diagnostic studies useful in evaluating older adults with somatic symptoms include urinalysis, serum electrolytes and glucose, calcium and vitamin D, renal and liver function tests, complete blood count, thyroid function tests, vitamin B_{12}, folate, syphilis serology, and medication levels as indicated. Other investigative recommendations are included in **Table 3**.

TREATMENT

About 70% of appropriately treated older adults recover from their first episode of late-life depression.[42] However, relapse rates tend to be higher when compared with younger patients. Several evidence-based pharmacologic and nonpharmacologic treatment modalities are available to treat late-life depression. Unless the patient requires urgent treatment (eg, acute suicidality, psychotic symptoms), the first step in management is to identify any underlying medical or situational factors that may be contributing to the patient's depression. This includes clinician efforts to discontinue medications that may be causing depression, resolving acute medical illness or chronic disease exacerbations, and exploring supportive strategies in the face of multiple losses.

There is no consensus regarding which treatment is most beneficial to older adults with depression. Both pharmacotherapy and psychotherapy may be considered as the first-line treatment. These may be used alone or in combination with each other.[43] When choosing a treatment, practitioners should elicit patient preference. This is especially relevant to older patients who may be more accustomed to a paternalistic rather than collaborative clinical approach. Although some data suggest this approach may be preferable to older patients,[44] age-associated differences in desire for decision-making involvement cannot be fully separated from psychological factors such as (depressed) mood and locus of control.[45] Optimal care thus requires accurate understanding of the whole patient including both medical and psychological factors. For patients who prefer collaboration, a shared decision-making (SDM) discussion

Table 2	
Medications that can cause symptoms of depression	
Analgesics	*Antiviral*
Narcotics	Zovirax
Antibiotics	*Cardiovascular*
Ciprofloxacin	Digitalis
Anticonvulsants	Diuretics
Celontin	Lidocaine
Zarontin	*Hypoglycemic agents*
Antihypertensives	*Hypnotics*
Angiotensin-converting enzyme inhibitors	Chloral hydrate
Calcium channel blockers (verapamil)	Benzodiazepines
Clonidine	*Psychotropic agents*
Hydralazine	Sedatives
β-Blockers (eg, propranolol)	Barbiturates
Reserpine	Benzodiazepines
Antimicrobials	Meprobamate
Sulfonamides	*Statins*
Isoniazid	Pravachol
Antiparkinsonism drugs	*Steroids*
Levodopa	Corticosteroids
Bromocriptine	Estrogens
Antipsychotics	*Others*
Chlorpromazine	Alcohol
Haloperidol	Chemotherapeutic agents
Thiothixene	Cimetidine

Data from Kotlyar M, Dysken M, Adson DE. Update on drug-induced depression in the elderly. Am J Geriatr Pharmacother. 2005;3(4):288-300.

should address the severity, duration, and type of the depressive episode; patient goals and preferences, cognitive function, socioeconomic status, contraindications to medication; and access to treatment.

Across all patient populations, a medicalized health-care system results in easier access to pharmacologic options despite health risks of geriatric polypharmacy[46] and calls for deprescribing by geriatric specialists.[47] In addition to safety concerns, some studies have indicated that medications may be less efficacious with increasing age and may not be consistent with patient preferences.[48–50]

In fact, a meta-analysis of nearly 69,000 patients of all ages found that 3 out of 4 preferred psychotherapy to medication although this trend seemed less clear among older adults.[51] Some data have shown that honoring patient preferences is insepa-rable from psychological treatment outcome.[52] Patients with impaired executive func-tion may also respond better to scheduled activities and psychotherapy than pharmacotherapy.

Table 3	
Diagnostic studies helpful in evaluating depressed geriatric patients with somatic symptoms	
Basic Evaluation	
History	
Physical examination	
Complete blood count	
Erythrocyte sedimentation rate	
Serum electrolytes, glucose, and calcium	
Renal function tests	
Liver function tests	
Thyroid function tests	
Calcium and vitamin D	
Serum B_{12} or methylmalonic acid	
Folate	
Syphilis serology	
Urinalysis	
Examples of other potentially helpful studies	
Symptom or sign	*Diagnostic study*
Pain	Evaluation for underlying cause (eg, appropriate radiological procedure such as bone fil, bone scan, GI series)
Chest pain	ECG, noninvasive cardiovascular studies (eg, exercise stress test, echocardiography, radionuclide scans)
Shortness of breath	Chest films, pulmonary function tests, pulse oximetry arterial blood gases
Constipation	Test for occult blood in stool, colonoscopy, abdominal radiograph, thyroid function tests
Focal neurologic signs or symptoms	CT or MRI scan, EEG

Abbreviations: CT, computed tomography; ECG, electrocardiography; EEG, electroencephalog-raphy; GI, gastrointestinal; MRI, magnetic resonance imaging.
From Chapter 7. Diagnosis and Management of Depression. In: Kane RL, Ouslander JG, Abrass IB, Resnick B. eds. Essentials of Clinical Geriatrics, 7e. McGraw Hill; 2013. Accessed October 20,2022. https://accessmedicine.mhmedical.com/content.aspx?bookid=678&sectionid=44833885.

Loneliness

Inseparable from aging and mood is loneliness, a key risk factor for morbidity and mortality among older adults.[53,54] Although not unique to aging, the health-related impact of loneliness can be particularly lethal in later life.[55] Clinically, it is important to differentiate loneliness, a subjective perception (ie, feeling), from isolation, an objective (quantitative) value for example, social network size, although both are often erroneously used and/or defined interchangeably.[56] Specific risk factors for loneliness include not being married/partnered and partner loss; a limited social network; a low level of social activity; poor self-perceived health; depressed mood, and an increase in depression.[57] Some data suggest loneliness and depression influence each other reciprocally.[58] Hearing loss among older adults has been associated with a 50% increased likelihood of loneliness[59] and increased odds of depression.[60] Clearly, ameliorating loneliness requires treatments that are customized more than standardized. The lack of a "one size fits all" approach makes evaluating comparative effectiveness among interventions difficult[61] and recent efforts to explicitly establish a standard framework for assessment and mitigation are underway.[62] Although potentially useful, loneliness, similar to other subjective emotions, is a direct treatment target of psychosocial intervention—be it individual or in a group—consistent with the notion that clinical opportunities for reminiscence and life review are therapeutic responses to universal aspects of the aging process.[63]

Psychosocial Treatments

Psychiatrist Robert Butler, who pioneered the National Institute of Aging and the nation's first academic department of geriatric medicine, deemphasized medicalizing elder care. Central to these efforts was Life Review, a reminiscence-oriented psychotherapy that targeted older adults' need for acceptance and closure toward the end of life.[64] Clinical efficacy of reminiscence therapy and other psychotherapeutic interventions targeting geriatric depression has been established for decades.[65–67] These include brief psychodynamic, interpersonal, and cognitive-behavioral therapy.[68] Supporting evidence includes group interventions[69] and group (ie, institutional) settings.[70] In addition to psychotherapeutic treatment, exercise programs have also been evaluated. A meta-analysis of exercise-based interventions (mind–body, resistance, aerobic) found superior efficacy of combined "mind–body" programs compared with control groups although no significant difference between exercise types.[71] Of course decreased motivation, a hallmark depressive symptom, makes engaging in exercise difficult, as do numerous aging-associated musculoskeletal conditions (eg, osteoarthritis) and well-established geriatric syndromes (eg, frailty, falls).[72] Efforts to link frailty and other geriatric syndromes with depression persist,[73] and antidepressant medication has been associated with increased fall risk.[74]

Pharmacotherapy

Depression is heterogeneous condition, which limits the ability to predict response and remission to antidepressant medications.[75] Pharmacotherapy should be considered when a patient meets criteria for major depression, is experiencing significant functional disability or difficulty recovering from other illness, or is not responding to nonpharmacologic interventions.

When selecting an antidepressant drug, the side effect profile must be carefully considered. Age-related changes in hepatic, renal, and gastrointestinal function may make older adults more susceptible to side effects, especially those affecting the central and autonomic nervous systems. Patients should be carefully monitored for sedation, anticholinergic effects, orthostatic hypotension, and extrapyramidal symptoms. These side effects are particularly hazardous because they could lead to falls and subsequent significant morbidity.

Multiple classes of medications are available and effective in the treatment of depression in older adults.[75] These include selective serotonin-reuptake inhibitors (SSRIs), tricyclic antidepressants (TCAs), monoamine oxidase inhibitors (MAOIs), and others. In general, studies have not shown significant differences in efficacy among various agents.[76,77] Therefore, the choice of pharmacotherapy depends on other drug and patient factors.

Selective serotonin reuptake inhibitors

Because of their more favorable side effect profile and affordability, SSRIs are the recommended first-line pharmacotherapy for late-life depression. There have been mixed results from randomized, controlled trials (RCTs). Some,[78–81] but not all,[82–84] RCTs demonstrate superiority of SSRIs over placebo in reducing symptoms of depression and increasing rates of remission. A recent systematic review found little evidence of an association between serotonin and depression but a potential correlation between increased antidepressant use and lower serotonin levels, underscoring the recognition of depression as a heterogenous condition that is unlikely to be linked to a single neurotransmitter.[85] The most frequently seen side effects among the various SSRIs include nausea, diarrhea, weight changes, increased risk of fractures (falls), sexual dysfunction, hyponatremia (particularly in women taking diuretics or low body mass index), and increased risk of gastrointestinal bleeding (especially when combined with nonsteroidal anti-inflammatory drugs or warfarin).[86] Sertraline and escitalopram are regarded as having the best safety profiles in older adults.[77]

Tricyclic antidepressants

TCAs are considered similarly effective to SSRIs in treating older adults with depression but are less well tolerated[87] and are included on the Beers list of potentially inappropriate medications in geriatric patients.[88] Of particular concern are their anticholinergic side effects including dry mouth, confusion, constipation, difficulty urinating, sedation, weight gain, and sexual dysfunction. They also have a quinidine-like effect that delays ventricular conduction. This class should be avoided in cognitively impaired patients. They may be considered in cases when other agents have not been effective. If considered, nortriptyline and desipramine are recommended based on their efficacy and side effect profiles. Nortriptyline is less likely to cause orthostatic hypotension than other TCAs, and desipramine is less sedating and thus more suitable for daytime use.[87]

Monoamine oxidase inhibitors

MAOIs may also be considered in the treatment of late-life depression. A small number of studies have demonstrated them to be safe and effective for use in older adults; however, in a literature review, it was concluded that more research was needed in geriatric patients and those with serious illnesses.[89] Their use is complicated by hypotension, hypertension, and food–drug interactions.

Other antidepressants

Serotonin-norepinephrine reuptake inhibitors are often used as second-line agents when remission is not achieved with SSRIs, although studies for their use in older adults is limited. The efficacy of venlaxafine has not been demonstrated in smaller studies but a larger study of duloxetine showed significant treatment response.[90] Blood pressure should be monitored when using venlaxafine in patients with cardiovascular disease or who are taking high doses.[77] Duloxetine is approved to treat depression and diabetic neuropathy but should not be used in patients with hepatic impairment.

The tetracyclic antidepressant mirtapazine is also used as a second-line agent. Although studies in older adults are limited, it may be useful in patients also suffering from anorexia or weight loss as well as in patients with insomnia, restlessness, or agitation.[91]

Titration and Monitoring

Clinical response to all classes of antidepressant medications may take longer in older adults and typically requires 2 to 6 weeks of therapy with remission requiring months.[87] Patients should be seen within 2 weeks of initiating medication so that concerns may be addressed and dose adjusted as necessary. Although lower starting doses are recommended in older adults, care must be taken to prescribe adequate therapeutic doses for a persistent amount of time. Therefore, dosing should be increased until the maximum dosage is reached, side effects limit further increases, or the patient experiences good symptomatic relief.[92] If a patient at the maximum dosage does not have adequate symptom relief after approximately 4 weeks, a different agent from the same or different class may be substituted, although in general the new agent should have a broader mechanism of action. In cases of partial response, the addition of a second class of medication (either another antidepressant or another adjunctive medication) can be considered although monotherapy is preferred.[77]

Because of progressively higher relapse rates after subsequent episodes of major depression, therapy should be continued for 1 year after remission after the first episode of depression, at least 1 to 2 years after a second episode, and 3 years after a third episode. Patients are particularly vulnerable in the first 6 to 12 months after remission and should be monitored monthly during that time and then every 3 months thereafter. If antidepressants are stopped, the dose should be tapered gradually while monitoring for relapse.[87]

Electroconvulsive Therapy

Electroconvulsive therapy (ECT) can be considered in older adults with depression and psychotic features who have not responded to pharmacotherapy or in patients with severe nonpsychotic depression who have not responded to adequate trials of multiple antidepressants. Patients are most likely to benefit from ECT if they suffer from delusions, early morning awakening, or if they have a family history of depression.[88] Although ECT can be an effective short-term therapy, it has higher relapse rates compared with other therapies. Long-term maintenance therapy may be required. In addition, it may be contraindicated in patients with recent myocardial infarction, brain tumor, cerebral aneurysm, and uncontrolled heart failure.[77] Evidence that ECT is superior to placebo is limited while memory loss due to ECT treatment is well-established,[93] causing some to recommend suspending ECT.[94] Others have criticized reliance on narrative reviews and subjective memory complaints.[95] Some data show subjectively reported memory improvement following ECT although this was associated with subjectively reported improvement in depression, as well, adding further complexity.[96] A new Cochrane Review of ECT for depression is forthcoming.[97]

BARRIERS TO DIAGNOSIS AND TREATMENT

Although patient-centered and evidence-based, there are still many barriers to optimal diagnosis and treatment of geriatric depression. Chief among them is the current structure of the United States health-care system, which separates rather than integrates medical, behavioral, and psychosocial health care. Care fragmentation and siloes persist despite decades-old arguments for biopsychosocial medicine and behavioral health care by physicians[98] and psychologists,[99] respectively. Integrated primary care from physicians and psychologists, especially suited to geriatrics,[100] is still not standard. A notable exception is the VA health system, which in 2007 began nationwide implementation of colocated primary care mental health integration[101] with a specific emphasis on collaborative depression care.[102] A recent analysis of associated utilization and costs found the VA integrated model successfully improved access to care at a cost increase of about 9% per patient per year.[103] Non-VA programs have demonstrated decreased costs from integrated primary care.[104] A direct cost comparison between second-generation antidepressants and cognitive behavioral therapy found that neither was consistently superior to the other although the authors reiterated patients' preference for psychotherapeutic treatment.[105]

SUMMARY

Late-life depression is a serious problem that requires mindful screening and assessment and watchful and persistent treatment when diagnosed. Although both pharmacotherapy and psychosocial treatments, or a combination of the two, are considered as the first-line therapy for late-life depression, most data support a combined, biopsychosocial treatment approach provided by an interdisciplinary team.

CLINICS CARE POINTS

- Depression is not a normal part of aging.
- Depression in older adults is often underrecognized and undertreated resulting in significant morbidity and mortality.
- Given the bidirectional relationship between depression and comorbidities in older adults, a careful history is essential in the diagnosis of depression.
- Suicide rates are highest in older adults and most older adults who commit suicide have seen a physician within the previous month.
- Late-life depression is treatable but older adults often take longer to respond to therapy and have higher relapse rates than younger patients. Older adults therefore benefit most from closely monitored, persistent care.
- Although both pharmacotherapy and psychosocial treatments, or a combination of the two, are considered as the first-line therapy for late-life depression, most data support a combined, biopsychosocial treatment approach provided by an interdisciplinary team.
- Patients should be assessed frequently after treatment of depression is initiated and after remission is achieved.

REFERENCES

1. Taylor. Depression in the elderly. N Engl J Med 2014;371:1228–36.
2. Lebowitz BD, Pearson JL, Schneider LS, et al. Diagnosis and treatment of depression in late life. Consensus statement update. JAMA 1997;278:1186.
3. Hybels CF, Blazer DG. Epidemiology of late-life mental disorders. Clin Geriatr Med 2003;19:663.

4. Valenstein M, Taylor KK, Austin K, et al. Benzodiazepene use among depressed patients treated in mental health settings. Am J Psychiatry 2004;161:654.
5. Unützer J. Clinical practice. Late-life depression. N Engl J Med 2007;357:2269.
6. Fyffe DC, Sirey JA, Heo M, Bruce ML. Late-life depression among black and white elderly homecare patients. Am J Geriatr Psychiatry 2004;12:531.
7. Crystal S, Sambamoorthi U, Walkup JT, Akincigil A. Diagnosis and treatment of depression in the elderly medicare population: predictors, disparities, and trends. J AM Geriatr Soc 2003;51:1718.
8. Unützer J, Katon W, Callahan CM, et al. Depression treatment in a sample of 1,801depressed older adults in primary care. J Am Geriatr Soc 2003;51:505.
9. Kessler RC, Birnbaum H, Bromet E, Hwang I, Sampson N, Shahly V. Age differences in major depression: results from the National Comorbidity Survey Replication (NCS-R). Psychol Med 2010;40(02):225–37 [PubMed: 19531277].
10. Jakobsen JC, Gluud C, Kirsch I. Should antidepressants be used for major depressive disorder? BMJ Evid Based Med 2020;25(4):130. Epub 2019 Sep 25. PMID: 31554608; PMCID: PMC7418603.
11. Butler RN. Age-ism: another form of bigotry. Gerontologist 1969;9(4):243–6.
12. Fiske A, Wetherell JL, Gatz M. Depression in older adults. Annu Rev Clin Psychol 2009;5:363–89.
13. Blazer DG. Depression in late life: review and commentary. J Gerontol A Biol Sci Med Sci 2003;58:249–65.
14. Alexopoulos GS, Katz IR, Reynolds CF, Carpenter D, Docherty JP. The expert consensus guideline series. Pharmacotherapy of depressive disorders in older patients. Postgrad Med 2001.
15. Cole MG, Dendukuri N. Risk factors for depression among elderly community subjects: a systematic review and meta-analysis. Am J Psychiatry 2003;160:1147.
16. Boswell EB, Stoudemire A. Major depression in the primary care setting. Am J Med 1996;101:3S–9S.
17. Blazer DG, Kessler RC, McGonagle KA, Swartz MS. The prevalence and distribution of major depression in a national community sample: the National Comorbidity Survey. Am J Psychiatry 1994;151:979.
18. Beekman AT, Geerlings SW, Deeg DJ, et al. The natural history of late-life depression: a 6-year prospective study in the community. Arch Gen Psychiatry 2022;59:605.
19. Suicide among older persons-United States, 1980-1992. MMWR Morb Mortal Wkly Rep 1996;45:3–6.
20. Bruce ML, Leaf PJ. Psychiatric disorders and 15-month mortality in a community sample of older adults. Am J Public Health 1989;79:727–30.
21. Ganzini L, Smith DM, Fenn DS, Lee MA. Depression and mortality in medically ill older adults. J Am Geriatr Soc 1997;45:307–12.
22. Waern M, Runeson BS, Allebeck P, Beskow J, Rubenowitz E, Skoog I, Wilhelmsson K. Mental disorder in elderly suicides: a case-control study. Am J Psychiatry 2002;159(3):450–5.
23. Hoyert DL, Kochanek KD, Murphy SL. Deaths: final data for 1997. Natl Vital Stat Rep 1999;47(19):1–104. PMID: 10410536.
24. Wiktorsson S, Berg AI, Wilhelmson K, Mellqvist Fässberg M, Van Orden K, Duberstein P, Waern M. Assessing the role of physical illness in young old and older old suicide attempters. Int J Geriatr Psychiatry 2016;31(7):771–4. Epub 2015 Nov 11. PMID: 26560405; PMCID: PMC4908825.

25. Reynolds CF 3rd, Dew MA, Frank E, et al. Effects of age at onset of first lifetime episode of recurrent major depression on treatment response and illness course in elderly patients. Am J Psychiatry 1988;155:795.

26. Schoevers RA, Geerlings MI, Beekman AT, Penninx BW, Deeg DJ, Jonker C, Van Tilburg W. Association of depression and gender with mortality in old age. Results from the Amsterdam Study of the Elderly (AMSTEL). Br J Psychiatry 2000; 177:336–42.

27. Cho HJ, Lavretsky H, Olmstead R, Levin MJ, Oxman MN, Irwin MR. Sleep disturbance and depression recurrence in community-dwelling older adults: a prospective study. Am J Psychiatry 2008;165(12):1543–50.

28. Diagnostic and statistical manual of mental disorders: DSM-5. 5th ed. American Psychiatric Association; 2013.

29. Mojtabai R. Diagnosing depression in older adults in primary care. N Engl J Med 2014;370:1180–2.

30. Crowley RA, Kirschner N, Health and Public Policy Committee of the American College of Physicians. The integration of care for mental health, substance abuse, and other behavioral health conditions into primary care: executive summary of an American College of Physicians position paper. Ann Intern Med 2015;163(4):298–9.

31. England MJ, Butler AS, Gonzalez ML, editors. Psychosocial interventions for mental and substance use disorders: a framework for establishing evidence-based standards. Washington, DC: National Academy Press; 2015. p. 57–69.

32. Li C, Friedman B, Conwell Y, Fiscella K. Validity of the Patient Health Questionnaire 2 (PHQ-2) in identifying major depression in older people. J Am Geriatr Soc 2007;55:596.

33. Montorio, Izal M. The geriatric depression scale: a review of its development and utility. Int Psychogeriatr 1996;8:103.

34. Rinaldi P, Mecocci P, Benedetti C, et al. Validation of the five-item geriatric depression scale in elderly subjects in three different settings. J Am Geriatr Soc 2003;51:694.

35. Hoyl MT, Alessi CA, Harker JO, et al. Development and testing of a five-item version of the Geriatric Depression Scale. J Am Geriatr Soc 1999;47:873.

36. Kroenke K, Spitzer RL, Williams JB. The PHQ-9: validity of a brief depression severity measure. J Gen Intern Med 2001;16:606.

37. Löwe B, Unützer J, Callahan CM, et al. Monitoring depression treatment outcomes with the patient health questionnaire-9. Med Care 2004;42:1194.

38. Alexopoulos GS, Abrams RC, Young RC, Shamoian CA. Cornell scale for depression in dementia. Biol Psychiatry 1988;23:271.

39. Kohout FJ, Berkman LF, Evans DA, Cornoni-Huntley J. Two shorter forms of the CES-D (Center for Epidemiological Studies Depression) depression symptoms index. J Aging Health 1993;5:179.

40. Radloff LS. The CES-D scale: the self-reported depression scale for research in the general population. Appl Psychol Meas 1977;1:385.

41. Haigh EAP, Bogucki OE, Sigmon ST, Blazer DG. Depression among older adults: a 20-year update on five common myths and misconceptions. Am J Geriatr Psychiatry 2018;26(1):107–22. Epub 2017 Jun 16. PMID: 28735658.

42. Bottino CM, Barcelos-Ferreira R, Ribeiz SR. Treatment of depression in older adults. Curr Psychiatry Rep 2012;14(4):289–97.

43. Areán PA, Cook BL. Psychotherapy and combined psychotherapy/pharmacotherapy for late life depression. Biol Psychiatry 2002 Aug 1;52(3):293–303. PMID: 12182934.

44. Murray E, Pollack L, White M, Lo B. Clinical decision-making: Patients' preferences and experiences. Patient Educ Couns 2007;65(2):189–96. Epub 2006 Sep 7. PMID: 16956742.
45. Schneider A, Körner T, Mehring M, Wensing M, Elwyn G, Szecsenyi J. Impact of age, health locus of control and psychological co-morbidity on patients' preferences for shared decision making in general practice. Patient Educ Couns 2006;61(2):292–8. PMID: 15896943.
46. Stevenson JM, Davies JG, Martin FC. Medication-related harm: a geriatric syndrome. Age Ageing 2020;49(1):7–11.
47. Garfinkel D. Poly-de-prescribing vs polypharmacy-the weapon to fight an iatrogenic epidemic: an overview. Eur J Geriatr Gerontol 2019;1(1):1–10.
48. Tedeschini E, Levkovitz Y, Iovieno N, Ameral VE, Nelson JC, Papakostas GI. Efficacy of antidepressants for late-life depression: a meta-analysis and meta-regression of placebo-controlled randomized trials. J Clin Psychiatry 2011; 72(12):1660–8. PMID: 22244025.
49. Gibbons RD, Hur K, Brown CH, Davis JM, Mann JJ. Benefits from antidepressants: synthesis of 6-week patient-level outcomes from double-blind placebo-controlled randomized trials of fluoxetine and venlafaxine. Arch Gen Psychiatry 2012;69(6):572–9. PMID: 22393205; PMCID: PMC3371295.
50. Robinson M, Oakes TM, Raskin J, Liu P, Shoemaker S, Nelson JC. Acute and long-term treatment of late-life major depressive disorder: duloxetine versus placebo. Am J Geriatr Psychiatry 2014;22(1):34–45. Epub 2013 Feb 6. PMID: 24314888.
51. McHugh RK, Whitton SW, Peckham AD, Welge JA, Otto MW. Patient preference for psychological vs pharmacologic treatment of psychiatric disorders: a meta-analytic review. J Clin Psychiatry 2013;74(6):595–602. PMID: 23842011; PMCID: PMC4156137.
52. Williams R, Farquharson L, Palmer L, Bassett P, Clarke J, Clark DM, Crawford MJ. Patient preference in psychological treatment and associations with self-reported outcome: national cross-sectional survey in England and Wales. BMC Psychiatry 2016;16:4. PMID: 26768890; PMCID: PMC4714467.
53. Ong AD, Uchino BN, Wethington E. Loneliness and health in older adults: a mini-review and synthesis. Gerontology 2016;62(4):443–9. Epub 2015 Nov 6. PMID: 26539997; PMCID: PMC6162046.
54. National Academies of Sciences, Engineering, and Medicine. Social isolation and loneliness in older adults: opportunities for the health care system. Washington, DC: National Academies Press; 2020.
55. Perissinotto CM, StijacicCenzer I, Covinsky KE. Loneliness in older persons: a predictor of functional decline and death. Arch Intern Med 2012;172(14): 1078–83. PMID: 22710744; PMCID: PMC4383762.
56. Courtin E, Knapp M. Social isolation, loneliness and health in old age: a scoping review. Health Soc Care Community 2017;25(3):799–812. Epub 2015 Dec 28. PMID: 26712585.
57. Dahlberg L, McKee KJ, Frank A, Naseer M. A systematic review of longitudinal risk factors for loneliness in older adults. Aging Ment Health 2022;26(2):225–49. PMID: 33563024.
58. Cacioppo JT, Hughes ME, Waite LJ, Hawkley LC, Thisted RA. Loneliness as a specific risk factor for depressive symptoms: cross-sectional and longitudinal analyses. Psychol Aging 2006;21(1):140–51.

59. Huang AR, Deal JA, Rebok GW, Pinto JM, Waite L, Lin FR. Hearing impairment and loneliness in older adults in the United States. J Appl Gerontol 2021;40(10): 1366–71. Epub 2020 Aug 4. PMID: 32749194.

60. Lawrence BJ, Jayakody DMP, Bennett RJ, Eikelboom RH, Gasson N, Friedland PL. Hearing loss and depression in older adults: a systematic review and meta-analysis. Gerontologist 2020;60(3):e137–54.

61. Fakoya OA, McCorry NK, Donnelly M. Loneliness and social isolation interventions for older adults: a scoping review of reviews. BMC Public Health 2020; 20:129.

62. Perissinotto C, Holt-Lunstad J, Periyakoil VS, Covinsky K. A Practical Approach to Assessing and Mitigating Loneliness and Isolation in Older Adults. J Am Geriatr Soc 2019;67(4):657–62. Epub 2019 Feb 14. PMID: 30762228.

63. Butler RN. Successful aging and the role of the life review. J Am Geriatr Soc 1974;22(12):529–35.

64. Butler RN. The life review: an interpretation of reminiscence in the aged. Psychiatry 1963;26:65–76.

65. Scogin F, McElreath L. Efficacy of psychocial treatments for geriatric depression: a quantitative review. J Consult Clin Psychol 1994;62(1):69.

66. Bohlmeijer E, Smit F, Cuijpers P. Effects of reminiscence and life review on late-life depression: a meta-analysis. Int J Geriatr Psychiatry 2003;18(12):1088–94.

67. Huang AX, Delucchi K, Dunn LB, Nelson JC. A systematic review and meta-analysis of psychotherapy for late-life depression. Am J Geriatr Psychiatry 2015;23(3):261–73. Epub 2014 Apr 23. PMID: 24856580.

68. Mackin RS, Areán PA. Evidence-based psychotherapeutic interventions for geriatric depression. Psychiatr Clin North Am 2005;28(4):805–20, vii-viiiPMID: 16325730.

69. Tavares LR, Barbosa MR. Efficacy of group psychotherapy for geriatric depression: A systematic review. Arch Gerontol Geriatr 2018;78:71–80. Epub 2018 Jun 18. PMID: 29933137.

70. Cody RA, Drysdale K. The effects of psychotherapy on reducing depression in residential aged care: A meta-analytic review. Clin Gerontol 2013;36(1):46–69.

71. Miller KJ, Gonçalves-Bradley DC, Areerob P, Hennessy D, Mesagno C, Grace F. Comparative effectiveness of three exercise types to treat clinical depression in older adults: A systematic review and network meta-analysis of randomised controlled trials. Ageing Res Rev 2020;58:100999. Epub 2019 Dec 11. PMID: 31837462.

72. Chen X, Mao G, Leng SX. Frailty syndrome: an overview. Clin Interv Aging 2014; 9:433–41. PMID: 24672230; PMCID: PMC3964027.

73. Borges MK, Oude Voshaar RC, Romanini CFV, Oliveira FM, Lima NA, Petrella M, Costa DL, Martinelli JE, Mingardi SVB, Siqueira A, Biela M, Collard R, Aprahamian I. Could frailty be an explanatory factor of the association between depression and other geriatric syndromes in later life? Clin Gerontol 2021;44(2): 143–53. PMID: 33100186.

74. van Poelgeest EP, Pronk AC, Rhebergen D, van der Velde N. Depression, antidepressants and fall risk: therapeutic dilemmas-a clinical review. Eur Geriatr Med 2021;12(3):585–96. Epub 2021 Mar 15. PMID: 33721264; PMCID: PMC8149338.

75. Masse-Sibille C, Djamila B, Julie G, Emmanuel H, Pierre V, Gilles C. Predictors of Response and Remission to Antidepressants in Geriatric Depression: A Systematic Review. J Geriatr Psychiatry Neurol 2018;31(6):283–302.

76. Mottram P, Wilson K, Strobl J. Antidepressants for depressed elderly. Cochrane Database Syst Ver 2006;1:CD003491.

77. Avasthi A, Grover S. Clinical practice guidelines for management of depression in elderly. Indian J Psychiatry 2018;60(Suppl 3):S341–62. PMID: 29535469; PMCID: PMC5840909.

78. Schneider LS, Nelson JC, Clary CM, Newhouse P, Krishnan KR, Shiovitz T, Weihs K. Sertraline Elderly Depression Study Group. An 8-week multicenter, parallel-group, double-blind, placebo-controlled study of sertraline in elderly outpatients with major depression. Am J Psychiatry 2003;160(7):1277–85. PMID: 12832242.

79. Sheikh JI, Cassidy EL, Doraiswamy PM, Salomon RM, Hornig M, Holland PJ, Mandel FS, Clary CM, Burt T. Efficacy, safety, and tolerability of sertraline in patients with late-life depression and comorbid medical illness. J Am Geriatr Soc 2004;52(1):86–92. Erratum in: J Am Geriatr Soc. 2004 Jul;52(7):1228. PMID: 14687320.

80. Raskin J, Wiltse CG, Siegal A, Sheikh J, Xu J, Dinkel JJ, Rotz BT, Mohs RC. Efficacy of duloxetine on cognition, depression, and pain in elderly patients with major depressive disorder: an 8-week, double-blind, placebo-controlled trial. Am J Psychiatry 2007;164(6):900–9.

81. Tollefson GD, Bosomworth JC, Heiligenstein JH, Potvin JH, Holman S. A double-blind, placebo-controlled clinical trial of fluoxetine in geriatric patients with major depression. The Fluoxetine Collaborative Study Group. Int Psychogeriatr 1995; 7(1):89–104.

82. Bose A, Li D, Gandhi C. Escitalopram in the acute treatment of depressed patients aged 60 years or older. Am J Geriatr Psychiatry 2008;16(1):14–20. PMID: 18165459.

83. Kasper S, de Swart H, Friis Andersen H. Escitalopram in the treatment of depressed elderly patients. Am J Geriatr Psychiatry 2005;13(10):884–91. PMID: 16223967.

84. Roose SP, Sackeim HA, Krishnan KR, Pollock BG, Alexopoulos G, Lavretsky H, Katz IR, Hakkarainen H. Old-old depression study group. antidepressant pharmacotherapy in the treatment of depression in the very old: a randomized, placebo-controlled trial. Am J Psychiatry 2004;161(11):2050–9.

85. Moncrieff J, Cooper RE, Stockmann T, Amendola S, Hengartner MP, Horowitz MA. The serotonin theory of depression: a systematic umbrella review of the evidence. Mol Psychiatry 2022. https://doi.org/10.1038/s41380-022-01661-0. Epub ahead of print. PMID: 35854107.

86. Solai LK, Mulsant BH, Pollock BG. Selective serotonin reuptake inhibitors for late-life depression: a comparative review. Drugs Aging 2001;18(5):355–68. PMID: 11392444.

87. Birrer RB, Vemuri SP. Depression in later life: a diagnostic and therapeutic challenge. Am Fam Physician 2004;69(10):2375–82. PMID: 15168957.

88. American Geriatrics Society 2012 Beers Criteria Update Expert Panel. American Geriatrics Society updated Beers Criteria for potentially inappropriate medication use in older adults. J Am Geriatr Soc 2012;60:616–31.

89. Salzman C, Wong E, Wright BC. Drug and ECT treatment of depression in the elderly, 1996-2001: a literature review. Biol Psychiatry 2002;52:265–84.

90. Nelson JC, Wohlreich MM, Mallinckrodt CH, et al. Duloxetine for the treatment of major depressive disorder in older patients. Am J Geriatr Psychiatry 2005;13(3): 227–35.

91. Anttila SA, Leinonen EV. A review of the pharmacological and clinical profile of mirtazapine. CNS Drug Rev 2001;7(3):249–64. PMID: 11607047; PMCID: PMC6494141.

92. Frank C. Pharmacologic treatment of depression in the elderly. Can Fam Physician 2014;60(2):121–6. PMID: 24522673; PMCID: PMC3922554.

93. Read J. response to yet another defence of ECT in the absence of robust efficacy and safety evidence. Epidemiol Psychiatr Sci 2022;31.

94. Read J, Kirsch I, McGrath L. Electroconvulsive therapy for depression: a review of the quality of ECT versus sham ECT trials and meta-analyses. Ethical Hum Psychol Psychiatry 2020;21(2).

95. Meechan CF, Laws KR, Young AH, McLoughlin DM, Jauhar S. A critique of narrative reviews of the evidence-base for ECT in depression. Epidemiol Psychiatr Sci 2022;31:e10. PMCID: PMC8851059.

96. Vann Jones S, McCollum R. Subjective memory complaints after electroconvulsive therapy: systematic review. Bjpsych Bull 2019;43(2):73–80. PMCID: PMC6472304.

97. Munkholm K, Jørgensen KJ, Paludan-Müller AS. Electroconvulsive therapy for preventing relapse and recurrence in people with depression. Cochrane Database Syst Rev 2022;1:CD015164.

98. Engel GL. The need for a new medical model: A challenge for biomedicine. Science 1977;196(4286):129–36.

99. Matarazzo JD. Behavioral health and behavioral medicine: Frontiers for a new health psychology. Am Psychol 1980;35(9):807–17.

100. Bensadon BA, editor. Psychology and geriatrics: integrated care for an aging population. Academic Press; 2015.

101. Johnson-Lawrence VD, Szymanski BR, Zivin K, McCarthy JF, Valenstein M, Pfeiffer PN. Primary care-mental health integration programs in the veterans affairs health system serve a different patient population than specialty mental health clinics. Prim Care Companion CNS Disord 2012;14(3):11m01286. Epub 2012 May 17. PMID: 23106026; PMCID: PMC3466035.

102. Chang ET, Rose DE, Yano EM, Wells KB, et al. Determinants of readiness for primary care-mental health integration (PC-MHI) in the VA health care system. J Gen Intern Med 2013;28(3):353–62.

103. Leung LB, Rubenstein LV, Yoon J, Post EP, Jaske E, Wells KB, Trivedi RB. Veterans health administration investments in primary care and mental health integration improved care access. Health Aff (Millwood) 2019;38(8):1281–8.

104. Ross KM, Gilchrist EC, Melek SP, Gordon PD, Ruland SL, Miller BF. Cost savings associated with an alternative payment model for integrating behavioral health in primary care. Transl Behav Med 2019;9(2):274–81.

105. Ross EL, Vijan S, Miller EM, Valenstein M, Zivin K. The cost-effectiveness of cognitive behavioral therapy versus second-generation antidepressants for initial treatment of major depressive disorder in the united states: a decision analytic model. Ann Intern Med 2019;171(11):785–95. Epub 2019 Oct 29. PMID: 31658472; PMCID: PMC7188559.

Moving?

Make sure your subscription moves with you!

To notify us of your new address, find your **Clinics Account Number** (located on your mailing label above your name), and contact customer service at:

Email: journalscustomerservice-usa@elsevier.com

800-654-2452 (subscribers in the U.S. & Canada)
314-447-8871 (subscribers outside of the U.S. & Canada)

Fax number: 314-447-8029

Elsevier Health Sciences Division
Subscription Customer Service
3251 Riverport Lane
Maryland Heights, MO 63043

*To ensure uninterrupted delivery of your subscription, please notify us at least 4 weeks in advance of move.